ADVENTURES OF A SURGICAL RESIDENT

ADVENTURES OF A SURGICAL RESIDENT

PHILIP B. DOBRIN, M.D.

ACKNOWLEDGMENTS

The author gratefully acknowledges the efforts of friends and colleagues who read some or all of the text. These people include Roger Hooverman, Bernard Marciante, Jim McFarland, and Joseph Balzano, M.D. But the author is especially grateful to Clarice Kieselburg who coordinated the preparation of the manuscript and Jean Airey who prepared the manuscript for publication.

CONTENTS

PREFACE

QUESTIONS AND ANSWERS ABOUT THIS BOOK

1. What is this book?

It is a memoir of the author's experiences as a surgical resident.

2. Who are the characters?

The stories and events described here are based on my recollections of real events. However, for the sake of privacy, the names of all the patients, doctors, nurses, and medical students have been fictionalized. Only the author's name remains unchanged.

3. Who may wish to read this book?

Those individuals who wish to consider a career in medicine, nursing, or other fields of health care. Also, those who see medical TV shows and want more insight into what really transpires in a hospital..

4. Will I be able to read and understand the text?

This book was written in plain, everyday English.

5. Will I be able to understand the new medical terms?

When the attending doctor or senior resident teaches something to the junior resident or medical student, you will be there and he or she will teach it to the reader as well.

***

After you have read this book, I'm sure you will agree that the lives of residents and the challenges they face are intense and very different from the romantic soap operas one sees on television.

Ooops, that's my pager going off. I've got to go.

CHAPTER 1

FIRST DAY

June thirtieth, nineteen seventy-five. It is six o'clock in the morning, and Lenny Goldstein and I stand at the main entrance to University Hospital. We are about to enter a new and exciting life. We are six weeks out of medical school; ready to begin a five year residency in General Surgery.

This is the first time I've met Lenny Goldstein face to face, but he has acquired an impressive reputation. Word has it that he reads every journal and textbook he can lay his hands on and remembers everything that he reads. I hate him!

Lenny is tall and gangly with a loping gait that makes him look like he doesn't have a worry in the world. He takes the stairs down to begin a three month rotation in the Emergency Department while I head to the third floor to join the General Surgery Service. As I start up the stairs, a young resident comes storming down at breakneck speed, his white lab coat billowing out behind him. He crashes into me.

"Code Blue," he shouts. "Cardiac arrest. Look out! Room 104. " He pushes me aside, and darts into a patient's room. He is followed by two other young doctors who seem to appear out of nowhere. All these young people are residents in training, doctors-to-be, and for the next five years, I will be one of them.

PHILIP B. DOBRIN, M.D.

CHAPTER 2

GENERAL SURGERY SERVICE

I join the General Surgery Service on the third floor. A *service* is a group of attending doctors, residents and medical students who work as a team. Dr. Peterson is the attending doctor on General Surgery. He is a fully-trained, experienced surgeon, and a master teacher of surgical judgment and technique. Ultimately, he is responsible for all the decisions we make, and the care we provide for his patients in and out of the operating room.

There are three residents on our service, including me. Our senior resident is Barney Wilson, a husky, soft-spoken Iowa farm boy who is in his fifth year. He is our on-field captain, the person who makes day-to-day decisions for patients out of the operating room. He also performs much of the surgery, assisting or sharing procedures with Dr. Peterson in the operating room.

Our third year resident is Nathan Forbes. He is short, wide and, to hear him tell it, a master of a large number of surgical procedures. Rumor has it that he will do almost anything to get to the cafeteria before it closes.

Finally, I am the first year resident. I have much to learn about the diagnosis and treatment of patients pre- and post-operatively, and I'm looking forward to getting some hands-on-surgical experience as well.

Two medical students, Ruth and Milton also are assigned to tag along with our service. They're here to learn, but they also help by performing *scut* work— calling the lab to obtain the results of blood tests, running down to Radiology to fetch x-rays, and entering daily notes in the charts. As the most junior resident with a state medical license, I am expected to read and countersign everything the medical students write in the charts.

****

The team is in the second floor nurses' station gathering up our patients' charts when Barney receives a call from Dr. Peterson. After a brief conversation, Barney alerts us to be on the lookout for someone named Edwin Hall. According to Dr. Peterson, Mr. Hall is a puzzle because he has two separate medical problems; a small aortic aneurysm, and also right groin pain that might be from a hernia. He is supposed to be coming in through the Emergency room. I write his name on a three-by-five card, and slip it into my pocket.

"Currently we have just three patients," Barney says, "Mr. Kazmarek, Mr. Finney and Mr. Cook. That's hardly a busy service, but the departing residents discharged everyone they could before they left for their next rotation."

Barney reviews the patients for us. "Mr. Kazmarek is a fifty-year old gentleman who is here for repair of a left inguinal hernia. Repair of hernias," Barney adds for the students, "Is one of the most frequently performed procedures that general surgeons do. Mr. Kazmarek first noticed discomfort and a bulge in the left groin while doing some home repairs. His family doctor referred him to Dr. Peterson."

Surgeons are different than internists and family practitioners in that surgeons don't have a regular stable of chronic patients that they follow the way internists do; they depend on referrals from internists and family practice doctors. After a surgeon has evaluated and possibly operated on a patient and the patient has

4

recovered, the surgeon sends him back to his referring physician.

We knock lightly on the door to Mr. Kazmarek's room, then push it open.

"Good morning," Barney announces to the patient. Mr. Kazmarek's eyes are open, but he doesn't seem to be awake. He blinks and surveys the five strangers in white lab coats crowding into his room.

"Good morning," Barney says again. "I'm Dr. Wilson; I met you in Dr. Peterson's clinic."

Mr. Kazmarek blinks without expression. According to his chart, the surgery resident who was on call in the hospital last night ordered something for sleep for Mr. Kazmarek. Evidently the medication is still effective.

"This is our service," Barney says as he points to the five of us.

Mr. Kazmarek nods.

"You will be our first case this morning, Mr. Kazmarek. A Transportation orderly will be here any minute to take you to the operating room."

Mr. Kazmarek slumps back down in his bed. Apparently he is too sleepy to rise, and is content to wait for Transportation.

We move on to the next patient, Mr. Finney. Barney introduces us to him. Mr. Finney is a thirty-five year old gentleman with an asymptomatic groin hernia. He wasn't aware of any problem until an internist discovered the hernia during a pre-employment physical. "Mr. Finney," Barney says, "You will be our second case this morning, but we have a few minutes now. Would you mind if our young doctors examined you?"

"Not at all," Mr. Finney says cheerfully. He seems to be pleased with all the attention he's receiving.

Barney pulls the privacy curtain to separate him from Mr. Kazmarek. Then he asks Mr. Finney to pull his pajamas down an inch or two to reveal his hernia. Mr. Finney stands at the bedside while Barney sits on the edge of the bed. For cleanliness, Barney puts a rubber glove on his right hand, and passes his index finger along Mr. Finney's thigh, his scrotum and his inguinal canal. The inguinal canal is a tunnel that permits blood vessels and nerves to pass between the abdomen and the leg.

Barney then asks Mr. Finney to turn away and cough.

Mr. Finney complies.

"I can feel an impulse when he coughs," Barney says. "Evidence of a hernia in the inguinal canal."

"Here," he adds, motioning to me and to the medical students. "Put a glove on and examine Mr. Finney."

I stand aside until both students have had a chance to examine the patient, then it's my turn. When Mr. Finney coughs; I clearly feel an impulse, a sensation of something in his inguinal canal, pushing outward against my finger tip, something being pushed by the pressure of the cough.

"There's your hernia," Barney says to Mr. Finney. "We'll see you in the operating room, about nine-thirty."

We proceed to our last patient, Mr. Cook. Barney tells us that five days ago, he and Dr. Peterson excised part of Mr. Cook's large intestine for cancer. He did not require a colostomy. We examine his incision, review his vital signs recorded by the nurses, and search through his daily lab reports. The nurse's entry in the chart tells us that he has had a small bowel movement, and that his urine is clean and uncontaminated. But Mr. Cook has a slight fever. Barney and the rest of us listen to his lungs, and urge him to take deep breaths. This requires discipline on his part because each breath pulls painfully on his abdominal incision. Barney says that Mr. Cook's slight increase in temperature may be due to accumulation of mucus secretions in his airway.

"Take this pillow," he says to Mr. Cook. "Pull it against your abdomen and let's hear a big cough."

Mr. Cook does his best, but his breaths and coughs are shallow. Barney also urges Mr. Cook to be up and about. It will make it easier to take big breaths.

"Philip," Barney says to me. "From now on, Mr. Cook is going to be *your* responsibility. You have to be

6

sure he gets up and walks around at least twice each eight hour shift. And while he's in bed, he uses that little plastic toy-like device that acts as an incentive for taking deep breaths. Use your stethoscope to listen to his lungs. Also, check his body temperature several times a day. We will expect a report from you whenever we make rounds."

When we return to the hall outside of Mr. Cook's room Barney addresses the students. "This fuss about coughing and clearing of the airway is no trivial matter. It would be a tragedy to have a patient undergo a successful operation, then succumb to an avoidable pneumonia."

"When do you think he will be able to go home?" one of the students asks Barney.

"When he is able to take solid food and keep it down, and when he has no fever. We also are waiting for the pathologist's report to tell us more about the tissue we removed. Also, we are going to have the oncologists see him before he leaves to see if they want to treat him.

As we leave Mr. Cook, I am struck by how much more there is to surgery than just cutting and sewing—fevers, diets, infections and more. And once a surgeon performs a procedure on a patient, he is responsible for him.

We return to the nurses' station to write orders and put notes in the charts when I hear rapid footsteps marching down the corridor. I look up to see a balding, middle-aged doctor in a gray lab coat. A black plastic name plate on his chest reads:

B. Peterson, M.D.

Attending, General Surgery

He is short, stands ramrod straight, and walks with a purposeful strut that tells the world that he abides no nonsense. A diminutive bald Napoleon, he is the indefatigable Dr. Peterson. He nods good morning to our group, and immediately, I feel a rise in tension in the nurses' station. "How is Mr. Cook's temperature and white count this morning?" Dr. Peterson asks.

I fumble for my three-by-five cards, but Barney is already there with an answer.

"His temp is exactly one hundred. Up from 98.6. I think it's pulmonary."

"And. . .?"

"We've got him on breathing exercises, and we have assigned our *crack* new junior resident to keep after him. If he doesn't improve by this afternoon, we'll get a chest x-ray."

"A *crack* new resident, eh?"

Peterson surveys our team, stopping when his gaze falls on me. "You're the new guy, right?"

"I am."

"Tell us, why are we so interested in Mr. Cook's temperature and white count?"

Before I can answer Dr. Peterson he reaches his hand out to me. "I'm Doctor Peterson" he says.

"Philip Dobrin. We shake hands. Dr. Peterson's grip is strong, but not crushing

"Welcome," he says. "Have you ever scrubbed on a hernia repair?"

"Last year, when I was a medical student."

"Do you remember any of it?"

"Some."

"Good. Have you reviewed hernia repairs in the textbook?"

"I have."

"Okay. You can observe us do Mr. Kazmarek, and then you can do Mr. Finney. Have you examined Mr. Finney?"

"Yes. This morning."

"What did you think?"

"I felt an asymptomatic hernia on the left, with a palpable impulse."

"What is an impulse?"

"A pushing sensation that you can feel from the outside when a person with a hernia strains. It is internal structures being pushed in the inguinal canal or through a weak area in the body wall."

"Very good." Peterson turns away, and starts toward the operating room.

Nathan lowers his voice, and leans toward me. "Those were good answers you gave Peterson. He gets here at five-thirty in the morning, and my guess is that he has all the information that he asks us for. I think he's testing us"

I check my watch. It's nearly 7:10; we're supposed to be in the operating room. As I hurry to the OR, I review the steps required to repair a hernia. They are unlike the neat pictures drawn in the textbooks, in real life, everything bleeds. I found that out right away. And the surgical repair can be more complicated than one might expect because the anatomy consists of several overlapping layers of tissue in several different planes. But it isn't rocket science. I can learn it.

This will be my first case. I'm looking forward to it, but I admit, I am anxious. Of course, I won't be there alone. Barney and Peterson will be there to help and guide me. I change into scrubs in the doctor's locker room, and head out to the operating room.

Who goes sailing by but Lenny Goldstein, weighted down by an armful of clean scrubs. "We've run short in the Emergency Room," he says.

So even Lenny Goldstein can be saddled with housekeeping chores. I'll bet even he will be jittery when he does his first hernia repair unless, of course, he knows all the important steps already.

PHILIP B. DOBRIN, M.D.

CHAPTER 3

IN THE OPERATING ROOM

As I hurry out of the locker room, I glance at myself in a full-length wall mirror. I see a lanky, ambitious young man who is not unlike all the other young surgical residents in the locker room. I enter the operating room at full speed where I crash into Dr. Peterson. He stares at me then turns to the large moon-like clock on the wall.

"Seven-seventeen," he says. "If you want to do surgery, you have to be here on time–seven-fifteen. If your first case is ten minutes late, then everybody will be ten minutes late throughout the day. That will cost the university thousands of dollars a year."

I get the message: I'm here by seven-fifteen, or Peterson will give my case away or do it himself.

***

The operating room is about the size of a large bedroom with white-tiled floors and walls. There is an adjustable operating table in the center of the room. Powerful OR lights are suspended over the operating table illuminating Mr. Kazmarek, who lies under a sterile paper drape. This completely covers him, except for the area where we are going to operate. Nathan scrubs the uncovered area with a solution that kills the bacteria that we all have on our skin.

A tape recorder somewhere in the room plays baroque keyboard music, Preludes and Fugues of Johann Sebastian Bach.

Nathan leans toward me. "I *hate* Peterson's music," he whispers. "It's so old-fashioned, I absolutely *hate* it. But he won't let us play anything else."

While we whisper, Peterson moves about the operating room until he's standing close behind us. "Bach builds character," he says in a voice filled with unshakeable conviction. "His music is an inspiration, and it has lasted for more than 300 years. Let's see how long your favorite group lasts. By the way, what is your current favorite group these days, the *Rancid Belly Button?*"

Everyone laughs, but it doesn't matter; Peterson is the boss, and what he wants to hear is what we all will hear.

After five minutes of scrubbing the abdomen, Peterson waves Nathan away. Then he nods to Dr. Hakeem, the anesthesiologist, to put Mr. Kazmarek to sleep. We watch him add several medications to the IV line until the patient relaxes and appears to be asleep. I have seen the anesthesiologists give medications to patients in the past, but I really don't know just what they are giving. One of these days I will have to look it up. When Dr. Hakeem tells us we can begin, we march out to the sink outside the operating room to scrub our hands and forearms for five minutes.

Peterson drops his scrub brush into the sink. We all do the same, and follow him back into the operating room.

There is one nurse in the room who is scrubbed, gowned and gloved, standing beside a tray of surgical instruments. She is prepared to closely assist the surgeon as he performs an operation. She's the *sterile scrub nurse.*

There is a second nurse in the room, who is also in scrubs. She is spotlessly clean, but she is not sterile. She is called the *circulating nurse.*

The *circulating* nurse is there to help us gown, glove, and deliver sterile instrument packs and sutures to the scrub nurse when she needs them for the surgeons.

She helps all of us wriggle into sterile gowns and gloves. Then we take our places at the operating table. Barney and Doctor Peterson stand opposite each other, one on each side of Kazmarek. Nathan and I also stand across from each other, but closer to the patient's feet. We are located where we can observe and hold instruments to retract the edges of the incision. Everyone but Barney and Peterson are here to learn, Barney and Peterson are here to repair the hernia and to teach.

Barney begins by making an incision over the hernia bulge, naming each anatomic layer as it comes into view. His voice takes on the monotone of a railroad conductor as he arrives at each station. Barney identifies a protruding hernia of soft tissue which he returns to its normal position in the abdomen. He repairs the floor of the defect, and strengthens it by applying a patch of screen door-like polypropylene mesh. Several times Barney asks for a particular surgical instrument. I reach up to pass it on, but the scrub nurse simply withholds it, sharply smacking the back of my hand. It is a statement that her relationship is with the surgeon, not with me, an intruding first year resident. It is also a signal that this is her domain and that she doesn't need any uneducated help. Finally, Barney closes the skin. He makes it all look so easy. There is no substitute for experience.

After Barney completes the repair, Dr. Hakeem, the anesthesiologist, terminates the anesthesia, and Mr. Kazmarek begins to awaken. We slide him onto a gurney brought beside the operating table, and we wheel him into the nearby Post Anesthesiology Recovery Room (PAR). There, recovery room nurses will monitor Mr. Kazmarek until he is fully awake.

Barney sits down at a counter in the PAR to dictate his operative report. It is a description of his findings and the operative procedures he performed. His operative report will permanently be in the medical record. He also writes postoperative orders—pain medications, directions to call our service if Mr. Kazmarek fails to urinate within four hours, and renewal of his regular blood pressure medications. While he is doing this, Nathan reviews with the medical students the procedure we just completed. I listen, soaking up all I can; I will be operating on Mr. Finney in just a few minutes, and I will need all the guidance I can get.

When we prepare to operate, we follow the standard operating room routine once again—wash our hands and forearms at the scrub sink, lightly shave the skin if it is necessary, paint and scrub the patient's abdomen with a sterilizing solution. Then we cover the patient with a sterile drape. All this is a routine that will be with me for all operations I will ever do.

After Mr. Finney is covered with a sterile paper drape, we take our places at the operating table. Dr. Peterson and I stand on opposite sides of the operating table. Then Dr. Peterson shows me exactly where to make the skin incision. My hand trembles as I pass the scalpel over the skin of a living human being, then clamp and awkwardly tie off some bleeding veins. Then I expose the open wound with a spreading instrument. I probe the depths of the opening searching for the strong, white tendonous fascia and red muscular layers that I learned in Anatomy class must be there. After I identify them I locate the hernia defect in the body wall and, using dissecting scissors, free it from the surrounding tissues.

Peterson directs my every move. "Be precise how you use those scissors," he warns me. "Watch the tips of your scissors, where they are going. Don't cut what you can't see."

Once I've identified the hernia, I use sutures to close the defect, and apply a non-absorbable polypropylene mesh to reinforce repair. It's like patching a screen door.

"Hold the forceps with your left hand," Peterson says. "And use them to pick up what you're going to sew. Grasp the needle holder with your right hand. Advance it, but rotate your wrist to follow the curvature of the needle; don't just force the curved needle straight through the tissues."

I am getting overloaded as Peterson's stream of instructions flows relentlessly.

"Be certain you can see what you're sewing," Peterson continues, "Watch what's *underneath* what you're sewing, wherever your needle is going."

I am struck by how this all seems like high stakes carpentry. Of course, there's more than two-by-fours riding on it. There's so much detail to know and attend to. I know I can do serious injury with the scalpel and scissors, but I feel protected by Dr. Peterson's watchful eye and directions. I suspect that the dissection skills I am learning today will be useful in *any* field of surgery.

I want to look like I know what I'm doing, but how can I? I'm just a rookie and everyone in the room knows it. I'm elated when I finish, convinced that I actually knew what I was doing . . . well, *most* of the time I did. I really couldn't do the operation by myself, but someday I will. It's a matter of identifying the anatomy and utilizing the surgical skills. I can't be expected to learn them all at once. I'll bet that even Lenny Goldstein won't know *exactly* what he's doing when he repairs his first hernia.

As I tie the knots to close the skin, Peterson quizzes the medical students, Ruth and Milton.

"What's the difference between a *direct* and an *indirect* hernia?" he asks. "You'd better look it up," he tells Ruth when she cannot answer.

"What's the difference between an *incarcerated* hernia and a *strangulated* hernia?" he asks.

Milton rambles a bit, but he cannot answer the question.

"You'd better look it up," Peterson says.

Is this Peterson's way of instructing the students, or his way of instructing me? In any case, I'm certainly going to look up the answers to those questions. The first time Peterson asks *me* a question I intend to know the answers.

I am buoyant as we slide Mr. Finney off the operating table, onto a gurney, and wheel him into the Recovery Room. I take a seat at a desk in the Post Anesthesia Recovery Room (PAR), from which I dictate my findings and description of the operation. It takes me a couple of false starts before I get the order of the steps remembered correctly. Then I write post-op orders, but I can't get over it—for the past forty-five minutes, I actually performed a real operation in a living person—with a little help, of course—okay with a *lot* of help.

CHAPTER 4

THE PUZZLING MISTER HALL

As I'm writing post-operative orders in the PAR, Dr. Peterson comes to me with an assignment, "Edwin Hall is here," he says, "In the Emergency Room. He's one of Dr. Benton's patients with a four centimeter aneurysm, and Benton thinks he might also have a hernia, but he's not sure. I'd like you to go down to the Emergency Room and see this patient. After you've examined him, give me a call and tell me what you found. Then I'll come down to see him for myself."

***

Mr. Hall is a slender, 50-year old gentleman who's complaining of pain in his left groin. According to what is written in his medical record, Dr. Benton, the Chief of Vascular Surgery, is following him for a small aortic aneurysm, a bulge of the artery wall. Aneurysms can rupture if they enlarge to six and a half or seven centimeters, but according to his medical record, Mr. Hall's aneurysm is only four centimeters. That's about the size of the normal aorta. It's almost unheard of for an aneurysm that small to rupture.

I examine Mr. Hall's groin and inguinal region for a possible hernia with new-found confidence. It was just half an hour ago that I grasped the same anatomic structures under direct vision in the operating room in

Mr. Finney. Now, examining Mr. Hall, I know *precisely* what I'm feeling. I press my finger up and into his inguinal canal.

"Turn your head, face away and cough," I say to Mr. Hall.

He complies.

Although I can't be sure, I think I feel a slight impulse on the left, a vague pushing sensation against my fingertip when he coughs, but it's not as certain as it felt in Mr. Finney.

I also feel the arterial pulses in Mr. Hall's femoral arteries. The arterial pulses feel normal; they might be diminished if the aneurysm were leaking.

When I leave Mr. Hall in the examining room to write my notes, I notice Lenny Goldstein sitting in the nurses' station with his nose in a book.

"Did you examine Hall?" I ask him.

"I did."

"What do you think?"

"It's the aneurysm." He doesn't look up.

"But it's only four centimeters. Too small to leak."

Lenny keeps reading.

"Why do you think it's the aneurysm?"

"Because I do."

"Because you do? That's it?'

I sit down to write my notes, when who comes strutting into the ER but Dr. Peterson. He gives me a big phony smile, like we're old war buddies who haven't seen each other since we fought together on the beach. He marches into the examining room to see Mr. Hall. After a few minutes, he emerges with a self- confident look.

"I detected an impulse on the left," he says. "And normal femoral artery pulses. It's hard to know for sure, but I think he may have a hernia."

"I found the same things," I tell him.

"Admit Hall to our service," Peterson says, "and order a barium enema for the morning. Maybe we'll be able to identify a hernia."

Peterson turns to Lenny and asks his opinion.

"I think it might be the aneurysm." Lenny answers. "I suppose it could be," Peterson answers thoughtfully. "But I don't think so. Benton's been following him for almost a year. He doesn't think it's the aneurysm or he would have repaired it. He's the chief of Vascular Surgery."

I'm thrilled; Peterson and I agree. The hell with smart-ass Lenny. I get a private room for Mr. Hall, and write admitting orders. Then I head back up to the floor.

At six o'clock, we make evening rounds. All of our patients are doing well. They are without wound problems or fevers or abnormal laboratory values. Mr. Finney, the man whose hernia I repaired this morning, has no swelling or excessive pain. Mr. Hall, our new admission, is also doing well, sitting up in bed, smoking a cigarette. We insist that he not smoke in bed, but he just laughs us off. I have a feeling that Mr. Hall is the self-indulgent sort who is going to smoke whenever and wherever he pleases. We finish rounds at six-thirty and, except for Nathan; we head home for the night. Nathan will remain in the hospital to take in-house calls.

As I drive out of the hospital parking lot, the reality of today's events hits me. Today I did my first real operation! I can't wait to tell my wife. Of course, she may not be interested in my accomplishments. She is as focused on her career as I am on mine. Hey! It's only six o'clock, early enough for me to see the kids before they go to bed. Maybe they would like to hear about my hernia repair. Of course, they are a little young for that.

PHILIP B. DOBRIN, M.D.

CHAPTER 5

MR. HALL EXPLAINED

The bedside alarm goes off at five-fifteen, and I'm back in the hospital by six o'clock. I'm ready for another day of it. Our service gathers for rounds, and we walk from patient to patient. I'm starting to feel comfortable with the routine. I write at full speed on my three-by-five cards: orders, labs, x-rays, results to be checked, consult requests to be written and sent. Now we have just a few patients, but what is this going to be like when we have ten or twelve?

When we get to Mr. Hall's room we knock lightly on his door, then push it open. Mr. Hall is lying in bed, on his back, the color of blue-white marble, cold to the touch. His eyes stare upward and unfocused. Barney thinks he's been dead for several hours, probably since the last time the night nurses checked on him. Barney telephones Peterson. He, like us, is stunned by the news.

"I'll talk to the family," Peterson says. "We have to get an autopsy."

We're all shocked. What could Mr. Hall have died from? He was a heavy smoker. Was it a heart attack? A pulmonary artery blood clot? That small aortic aneurysm?

We finish morning rounds, then the team heads for the operating room for this morning's cases. All except me. Peterson sends me down to the morgue to observe the autopsy and report back what is found. He was *my* patient, and I'm brimming with curiosity. I'm pleased that Peterson selected me to watch the autopsy. Dr. Benton, the Chief of Vascular Surgery, is also there. He nods, "Good morning," but otherwise keeps to himself.

The morgue is in the basement, a locked room with a heavy steel door, back behind the loading dock. It's a chilly, hollow place with pale green tile walls and a white tile floor. A mop and a dented galvanized metal pail sit in the corner. The room is filled with the pungent smell of Lysol. Two stainless steel tables, the size of gurney stretchers, are in the middle of the room, and Mr. Hall lies stone-white on one of them, his eyes rolled back in his head. He's completely naked, and I have an irrational urge to cover him. It's so cold down here, and it seems immodest for him to be completely exposed.

At eight o'clock the pathologist arrives. Dr. Benton and I wrap ourselves in full-length black plastic aprons, put on surgical caps, masks and plastic goggles, and move close to the table to watch the autopsy. The pathologist is a bald, bullet-headed man named Bruno. With a single dispassionate slash of a scalpel, he opens Mr. Hall's abdomen from the lower margin of the ribs to the superficial regions of the pelvis.

"Let's see what we find here." Bruno's words are laced with a strong Bulgarian accent

"Aha," he says with morbid delight.

There is no hernia, but there's an unmistakable pool of dark, stagnant blood tracking from the abdomen down into the left groin, and in the center of the pool is a small, ruptured aortic aneurysm.

Damn that Lenny. He was right.

I leave the morgue to report what I have seen. But before I join Dr. Peterson and our service in the operating room, I stop off in the ER to tell Lenny what we found.

"Doesn't surprise me," he says with smug indifference.

22

"Why did you think it was the aneurysm?"

"He had a known diagnosis that would account for his symptoms—the aneurysm. He didn't need a diagnosis of a second illness."

"But Benton and Peterson both examined him."

Lenny shrugs. "The rupture rate for that size aneurysm is probably very low," he says. "But it's not zero."

I can't argue with that. I leave Lenny, and head up to the operating room.

Peterson's in the middle of an operation, deep in the abdomen.

"It was that small aneurysm," I tell him. "It bled and drained down into his groin."

"No shit," Peterson says without looking up." He clamps, cuts and ties a small blood vessel. "Did you tell Benton?"

"He was there, at the autopsy."

"He was! What did he have to say?"

"He didn't say anything, not to me anyway."

23

CHAPTER 6

NIGHT CALL

It is six-thirty, and we are ready for morning rounds. But today there is no rush. We don't have surgery scheduled for this morning, and at nine o'clock we are to join Dr. Peterson in his morning clinic.

We make inpatient rounds at a leisurely pace, visit each patient, inspect their surgical incisions, and review their vital signs and lab data. We write discharge orders for Mr. Kazmarek and Mr. Finney, the patients whose hernias we repaired yesterday.

"The time is coming," Barney says, "when we'll be doing these procedures on an outpatient basis. I predict that we'll do the surgery in the hospital, then send the patients home the same day. The problem is going to be for those patients who have no one at home to care for them during the recovery period. And it will be a real problem for indigent patients who have nowhere to sleep but under the viaduct." He shrugs. "But that's a problem for the administrators to solve."

Our last patient is Mr. Cook the genial sixty-five year old gentleman from whom Dr. Peterson removed a segment of large intestine for colon cancer. Today is Mr. Cook's sixth postoperative day. He's made excellent clinical progress, his wound looks clean and dry, he has no fever, and his lab data are normal. His lungs sound clear, and his cancer appears to be well-contained. We are waiting for the oncologists to see him and suggest a regimen of chemotherapy. As soon as they see him and put a note in his chart, we'll send him home.

We finish morning rounds at eight-thirty, then stroll over to the cafeteria for an unexpected treat—breakfast. We all have coffee except for Nathan, our always-hungry third year resident. Nathan buttons up his white lab coat, and orders bacon and eggs and a grease-ladened donut.

"He's always preaching to patients about avoiding high-fat foods and following the rules of healthy living," Barney says. "But apparently he doesn't listen to his own advice. All he needs now is a cigar to achieve complete hypocrisy."

That gets a laugh from our medical students.

"I hardly ever eat breakfast," Nathan insists. "Maybe once a year."

"Right," Barney says. "That's what you said last week."

Nathan shrugs as he crunches his way through a mouthful of crispy bacon.

After we finish eating, we sit in the cafeteria for a few quiet moments before heading off to clinic.

"I'm curious," Ruth says. "Do many residents view surgery as a desirable specialty to go into?"

"Oh, yes," Barney says. "It's very competitive. The work is challenging, and the income is good, although the hours can be demanding, especially if you're a woman trying to raise a family. Still, I couldn't imagine being a family practitioner or an internist, seeing the same group of patients in the outpatient clinic, day in and day out, six days a week.

Ruth nods. "So I guess a lot of medical students apply to surgery training programs?"

"You bet they do. We have eight slots for each year."

"Peterson told me that we had more than eight hundred applications for those eight positions, although most students apply to several different programs at once."

Ruth shakes her head in disbelief. "Eight hundred applications! How do they decide who to take?"

"Those who get good grades in medical school. They also like people who are going to remain in academic surgery, people who will publish research papers. It brings prestige to the department."

"What do you guys plan to do when you finish?" Milton asks.

"When I finish," Barney says. "I'm going to do a fellowship in vascular surgery—one year in the lab, a second year doing clinical work. My wife isn't happy about two more years of training, but it's a good career move. It's easier to keep up to date if you have a limited field to cover."

I have to admire him. That's two extra years of training after five years of general surgery residency, after four years of medical school, after four years of college. Wow!

Nathan gulps some scalding coffee. "My father's a general surgeon in Iowa," he says. "I'm going to join him as a partner. In any case, he's planning to retire in a couple of years, and I will either buy or inherit the practice from him."

This is something we don't usually talk about—the business side of medicine.

"How about you?" Ruth and Milton ask, turning their attention to me.

"Well, I'm just beginning," I say. "I'm interested in General Surgery, but I'll probably stay in an academic position like here where I can see patients, do some teaching and also do research. I have to admit it: I am fascinated by the unsolved problems in Medicine and Surgery. I feel certain that we can improve what we do for patients."

Milton yawns. He's not impressed. In any case, these decisions are years away for him, but he'll be facing them before he knows it.

It's ten minutes to nine and we're off to the clinic. As we begin walking, Barney explains to us how things work. "We usually have twenty-five to thirty scheduled patients, plus a few add-ons. We see each patient before Peterson meets them; we get their medical history, examine them and make a tentative diagnosis. Then we accompany Peterson when he goes into the examining room to see each patient for himself. If the patient has pathology that requires surgery, Dr. Peterson explains it to them in simple language. Some patients say yes right then and there; but most want to think about it, or get a second opinion."

"By the way," Barney says. "A word of caution. Never take a medical history or examine a female patient without a female nurse in the room with you."

Each student nods for a moment as they imagine the worst of possibilities.

We reach the examining room and meet our first patient.

"Mrs. Luchetti," Dr. Peterson says to an overweight middle-age lady with documented diabetes. "We have the results of the sonogram we performed last week. As we suspected, the test shows that you have stones in your gall bladder. That's why your abdomen hurts after you eat a large, fatty meal."

I don't think Mrs. Luchetti understands everything that Dr. Peterson explains, but she nods knowingly.

"What can you do for it?" she asks. "Are there medications I can take?"

"I'm afraid not," Peterson says. "There are some procedures we can do, but the stones can come back; only surgery can provide a cure. We remove the gall bladder with the stones. It's called a cholecystectomy—a very common operation. We do a lot of them.

Mrs. Luchetti bites her lip, her eyes fill with tears.

"So there's nothing that works as well as surgery?"

"I'm afraid not."

"How long would I be in the hospital?" she asks.

"Oh, four to six days."

"Would it be painful?"

"For a few days. Post-op pain, where we make the incision. But we would treat you with pain medication."

"Well," she says reluctantly. "I'd like to think about it."

"Certainly," Dr. Peterson says, "But I wouldn't put it off for too long. You're bound to have more attacks. If the gall bladder perforates and leaks bile, you will be very sick. And the fact that you have diabetes may increase your risks."

Mrs. Luchetti nods, half-listening, eyes glistening with sequestered tears, as she contemplates the prospect of undergoing surgery.

Urging a patient to undergo a procedure can be a problem for the surgeon who knows the medical risks of waiting versus not waiting. He wants to do what is best for the patient, but he does not want to press the issue. This not a life/death decision at this time, and it may never become so. But when we assemble in the hall outside the examining room Peterson says candidly, "She will be back, you'll see."

We see a continuous stream of patients until we have examined 28 of them, an honest day's work.

"Oh, damn," Nathan says as he looks at his watch. "With all this talking, I missed lunch hour in the cafeteria."

There is a mock outpouring of sorrow for poor starving Nathan, but none of us feels the slightest bit sorry for him.

"You've had enough fat for the entire service," Barney says. "I figure that one of these days we're going to be doing your gall bladder."

Nathan waves us away; he is a man who doesn't want to think about biliary stones and gall bladder disease.

***

It's a quiet afternoon, leaving time to do some paperwork and dictate the Discharge Summaries for the patients we've sent home. I walk downstairs to the lower level to the Medical Records Department. There I find a sagging shelf that seems to be as long as a football field. It is filled with medical records grouped by the resident who is responsible for their completion. My charts are there, on the ten yard line.

I pull out the two charts assigned to me, find a closet-sized cubicle that is lined with sound-deadening panels, and pick up the dictation telephone.

A discharge summary is a brief description of each patient's course while he or she was in the hospital. The summaries need only be one or two pages long, but they require that we go through the patient's chart to reconstruct the key steps in their care.

Discharge summaries are our introduction to the growing burden of paperwork overtaking all of medicine. The Summaries and Medical records (the patient's chart) must be completed with every entry signed and dated by an attending or resident physician. This is mandatory if the hospital and Dr. Peterson are going to be paid by the insurance companies. Federal agencies like Medicare and state agencies like Medicaid also require them to be completed. It's not surprising that completed Discharge Summaries are near and dear to Dr. Peterson's heart and to the hospital administrator's pocketbook.

If we fail to keep up with our Discharge Summaries and medical records, hospital administration will come after us; we may be temporarily banned from the operating room, or we may be required to take forced vacation days to complete the summaries, or we may even be subject to the withholding of our paychecks. The legality of withholding our paychecks is before the courts; hospitals really can't make people work without a salary. For surgical residents, banishment from the operating room usually is incentive enough.

So I begin to summarize the patient's care. It's Mr. Kazmarek, the gentleman whose hernia Barney and Peterson repaired yesterday. It will take me a few minutes to pull the information I need out of the chart, but it should be easy. After that, I will have to dictate Mr. Finney's discharge summary. After I've completed the discharge summaries, I may get a chance to slip away to read the textbook and some journal articles about gall bladder disease. From what I've heard, that's how Lenny Goldstein does it. He's never without a book.

***

We make evening rounds at five o'clock. Afterward, Nathan and Ruth head for the parking lot, leaving Milton and me alone on call. My first night on call—it's unsettling because I will be alone making all the clinical decisions. I remember the feeling as a medical student; you never know what you're going to encounter when the pager goes off.

"Philip," Barney says before leaving. "Do your best, but don't just wing it. If you're not sure what to do, call me. No matter how late it is, or how trivial the problem, or how many times you have to call me, do so. I'll sleep a lot better if I know you'll call me when you are not sure what to do."

Frankly, I am embarrassed, but Barney's words are reassuring.

Let me see, I think to myself; every third night for the next five years, that's six hundred nights of sleeping in the hospital ... no, it's six hundred nights of *not* sleeping in the hospital.

Before beginning our evening's work, Milton and I visit the cafeteria for a dose of meat loaf. "Dinner therapy," Milton calls it.

Afterwards, we start the evening's admissions, the patients coming in tonight for elective surgery tomorrow. "You'd better write a list of what we have to do," I tell him. "We're responsible for all the patients coming into General Surgery, Plastic Surgery and Vascular Surgery."

"I thought being a resident was going to be dramatic," Milton says. "Like on television with all kinds of life and death action."

"Sorry, it's a lot of paperwork with a variety of life and death forms. And it really is life and death." I tell him. "If we forget to complete all those forms or fail to include them in the patient's chart the operation will be delayed or even cancelled and the attending will kill us."

Milton laughs, but it's no joke; the patient's insurance will not pay for an extra day of in-house admission when absolutely nothing critical was done.

"When I was a medical student," I tell him, "one of the residents failed to include some paperwork and the

31

operation was cancelled. It was an honest mistake, but he really paid for it. Let's just say that, currently, he is in another field of medicine."

Milton shakes his head in disbelief. "Where did all this paperwork come from?"

"You can thank the Informed Consumer Movement for much of it, the Joint Commission, a group that evaluates hospitals, and don't forget the lawyers. You must always include the lawyers."

"All right," I say to Milton. "I'll take the first two patients, you take the next two."

By ten o'clock we have taken care of all our admissions. I sign Milton's entries in his charts, and we withdraw to the call rooms.

But before we leave, Milton asks, "Why is it that residents work such long hours, day after day? You hear all those horror stories of residents who go for weeks without sleep. Even if they are exaggerated, wouldn't they be better off if they just worked a regular eight hour shift?"

"Yes," I tell him. "They might be better off, but many of the spokesmen for the Medicine and Surgery training programs say that the long hours are desirable because they guarantee continuity of patient care. That is a potentially greater problem for surgery than it is for the noninvasive specialties because one team is present for the pre-op, operative and post-op care. That would get watered down if the residents changed every eight hours."

Milton mulls over my explanation.

"But in the end," I say. "This may be simpler than all that because hospitals have to pay the residents' salaries and that may be the crucial issue—who is going to pay the extra residents' salaries? It is estimated that the increase in residents' time would cost millions of dollars.

After I am convinced that Milton is suitably confused, I encourage him to study and sleep, and I promise to wake him if there's anything interesting to see. I retreat to my call room, and wait for the pager to go off. It will. Eight and a half hours is too long to not have lots of pages and phone calls.

At midnight, I am called by a nurse to see an elderly lady who fell and struck her head while getting out of the hospital bed. I awaken Milton, and we walk down together to examine the woman. She's a feisty, gray-haired lady in her eighties, in the hospital for a urological procedure to be performed in the morning.

"No," she insists. "I did not lose consciousness. Yes, of course I know where I am. I'm in the hospital. Yes, of course I know who the president is. It's Gerald Ford, but I'm not going to dignify that bunch in Washington by talking about them. You can't trust any of them. . ."

I ask Milton to perform a brief neurological examination on her, and then put a brief note in her chart. I ask the nurse to rouse the patient in three or four hours to be sure she can be awakened. "Bleeding in the skull puts pressure on the brain, and that leads to trouble," I tell Milton. "Making sure she can be awakened and that she has normal pupillary eye responses is an easy way to assess her."

I finish my note, and we return to the call rooms. "Let's see if we can get some sleep," I tell Milton. "You never know when a patient may show up with something serious."

CHAPTER 7

INCARCERATED HERNIA

It is 4 a.m. when I am awakened by a call from the doctor working in the Emergency Room asking me to come down to see a 66 year old gentleman with a possible incarcerated hernia. I awaken Milton, then review the various types of hernias as we descend the stairs.

"Most hernias can be reduced or pushed back into the abdomen," I tell him. "But an incarcerated hernia is one that is caught in the inguinal canal or in an opening in the abdominal wall, and it cannot be pushed back in. Think of an incarcerated hernia as one that is imprisoned.

"A strangulated hernia is different; it is a hernia that has been caught and is twisted, impairing its blood supply. This puts the tissue at risk because tissue can't live without an adequate blood supply. We repair incarcerated hernias urgently to prevent them from becoming strangulated, and we repair strangulated hernias promptly to avoid returning dead or dying tissue into the abdomen."

"Got it," Milton says.

In Emergency Room One, we find Mr. Sorenson, a sleek, silver-haired sixty-six year old gentleman with a slightly tender, lemon-size bulge in his right groin. He tells us that the bulge has been present for several months, but that it always disappeared when he lies down. Since midnight, however, the bulge has remained, and has become increasingly tender. Clearly, he has a right inguinal hernia that is incarcerated and cannot slip back into the abdomen. Hopefully, it is not strangulated. I place a stethoscope over the bulge, and I can hear bowel sounds. That suggests that the bulge includes a loop of intestine. Mr. Sorenson's temperature and white blood count are normal. That's the good news. I would expect them to be markedly elevated if the trapped intestine were strangulated and deprived of its blood supply.

After examining Mr. Sorenson, I telephone Barney. He answers on the first ring and seems completely awake. Remarkable, but I guess he's been doing this for a few years.

"Is it tender?" he asks.

"Not really. I can press gently on the mass, and the patient doesn't seem to mind."

"Are you sure it's incarcerated?"

"Well, I pressed on it, but I can't reduce it. I can't push it back in."

"Well, don't overdo it or you'll injure whatever is trapped in there." Barney warns. "You never want to force dead bowel back into the abdomen, or we'll really have our hands full. How about his temperature and white count?"

"His temp and white blood cell count are only slightly elevated. Doesn't sound strangulated to me."

"All right," he says. "It's four-thirty. Admit him, get all his lab work and paperwork done, have the anesthesiologist on call in the hospital see him, and we'll do him first case in the morning. Call the OR to let them know. And you had better call Peterson, also. Tell him you spoke with me and our plan to do him first case."

"Okay"

"I really should come in to see him," Barney says. "But it sounds like you are on top of it; besides, it's only a couple of hours before we'll be making rounds."

What he says is encouraging. It sounds like he has confidence in me.

"One more thing," he adds, "when you get this guy upstairs, put him in bed, and raise the lower part of the bed to get gravity working for you. The hernia may reduce on its own. Give him a little Valium to relax his abdominal wall musculature. And you might try putting a lightweight ice bag on the mass. That often works in kids. But whatever you do, don't force the mass back in or you could force a loop of dead bowel back into the abdomen. That's the worse thing you could do."

I go over everything with Milton, and teach him with a confidence and self-assurance that belies the fact that I just learned it all myself. We get Mr. Sorenson's signature on the various surgical consent forms, start an IV in a vein in his arm, and I get on the phone to get things rolling. I call the anesthesiologist, the OR scheduling desk, and Dr. Peterson.

"This is going to be great," Milton says. "I can't wait to see what it looks like from the inside, from the abdomen."

"Me, too."

"We won't have long to wait, just an hour or two."

***

We start morning rounds at six-thirty where we are joined by Katie, the head nurse on the surgical patients' floor. It's helpful when informed nurses accompany us because often they have information to share about the patients. Even as a medical student, I was struck by the fact that doctors focus on patients' diseases, whereas nurses know more about their patients as people.

Morning rounds go smoothly. When we come to Mr. Sorenson, I proudly present him to the team as though he were my personal property. I'm gratified when Barney and Dr. Peterson examine him, and both agree with my diagnosis. While we are discussing his case a Transportation Department orderly arrives with a gurney to take Mr. Sorenson to the operating room. I'm eager to get going too.

The last patient we see this morning is Mr. Cook He is the gentleman Dr. Peterson operated on six or seven days ago to remove a segment of his bowel for cancer. We met on my first day on the service, and I was assigned the task of keeping his lungs clear. Katie tells us that he has done well through the night, and his breath sounds are much improved. He is tolerating solid food. His vital signs are normal. A consult from the oncologists is in the chart; they will arrange to give him intravenous 5-fluorouricil chemotherapy on an outpatient basis. Dr. Peterson and Barney agree that he's ready for discharge. Katie says that his family is staying at a nearby motel, and they should be here at seven-thirty.

After we've seen Mr. Cook, the group breaks up and heads to the operating room.

"Before you go," Katie says, taking my arm. "How about writing Mr. Cook's discharge orders?"

I check my watch——seven-ten. "I can't," I tell her. "I've got to get to the Operating Room by seven-fifteen or Peterson will give my case away."

"It won't take that long," she says. "The family will be here any minute, and they've got a long drive, out of state." She looks at me earnestly, acting as a patient advocate.

How can I say no? "Well, I'll see what I can do. But I can't be late."

I write discharge orders in the chart:

Home today. Return to Surgery clinic in one week for follow-up

Return to Oncology Clinic in three weeks

Philip Dobrin, MD

My watch says seven-twelve.

I grab a handful of blank prescription forms, review Mr. Cook's medication profile, and start writing prescriptions——medications for post-op pain, for high blood pressure, for diabetes, for arthritis. Faster! Faster! What have I forgotten? I hand them to Katie.

Seven-fourteen

I race down the hall to the operating room, tear off the scrubs I've been wearing all night, change into fresh ones and dash into OR Room Six. Barney, Nathan, Peterson, and the medical students are all standing there, waiting for me. They are gowned and gloved and, ready to go. Wait, this is my case!

Dr. Peterson glares at me over his surgical mask, and glances at my old adversary, the moon-like wall clock.

"Seven-nineteen," he announces. "Nathan will do the case."

Milton shoots a sympathetic glance in my direction, but it doesn't help.

I am disappointed—seven-nineteen—four lousy minutes late to save Mr. Cook's family an hour and half of waiting, and Peterson is acting like Hitler. After I made the diagnosis and was up all night doing scut work while they were able to sleep.

Nathan is starting to make the incision, so I do my best to set my resentments aside. I move up to the operating table to stand directly behind Nathan, and observe over his shoulder. I watch him pass the scalpel lightly over the bulge, just enough to incise the skin. I can almost feel the coolness of the scalpel in my hand. After he incises the skin, he uses curved Metzenbaum scissors to carefully dissect the superficial bands adherent to the bulging incarcerated mass. It's like a lemon protruding upward, stuck to the skin that covers it, and bound by the superficial bands of muscle and fascia that are beneath and beside it.

I still can't tell what it is with certainty, but it sure looks like a loop of intestine, swollen and edematous. If Nathan makes a hole in it, bowel contents will come spilling out, bathing the wound with millions of bacteria; this will almost certainly cause a wound infection, destroying Nathan's repair. Nathan must free the incarcerated mass, but he must not injure it or let it fall back into the abdomen.

Peterson looks at Nathan. "This part can be tricky," he says. "Why don't you let me work on it for a while?"

That's the last time Nathan will see those scissors, I think to myself.

Reluctantly, Nathan gives up the scissors. Peterson begins cautiously to free the incarcerated mass. After a few minutes of meticulous dissection, we can see that the mass is bowel, that it is fully mobile, intact and uninjured. Peterson says "au revoir" to the mass with a playful wave as he drops it back into the abdomen. His speech is a poor excuse for a French accent. His "au revoir" gets a laugh, but it isn't funny—he stole my case.

I'm not sure how I feel about Peterson. Mr. Sorenson was my patient, not his, and although Peterson stole my case, I have to admit that he did a brilliant job of dissecting without injuring the bowel.

Now he gives the curved scissors back to Nathan. From that point on, the case proceeds as a routine hernia repair, closing the fascia and muscular defects, and applying a mesh patch, just as I did on Mr. Finney, two days ago.

I leave the operating room and return to the floor. What a great case, but I'm still fuming about how it was taken away from me, just because I was a lousy four minutes late to the OR—and all to keep Mr. Cook and his family from having to wait for an hour and a half. Maybe next time I'll let the departing patient wait, or I'll ask someone else to write the discharge orders.

When Mr. Sorenson is in the recovery room, Barney and I slip away to the cafeteria for a cup of coffee. We find a table in the corner where we can be by ourselves.

"Nice diagnosis on Sorenson," he says.

"Thanks. As soon as I saw him in the ER, I knew it was incarcerated."

"I had one of those when I was a first year," Barney says. "A difficult incarcerated groin hernia. Really stuck. Surrounded by scar tissue. A lot worse than Sorenson. I didn't know how we were going to free it up."

"Yeah. But at least you got to do your own case."

"Oh no," Barney says. "Peterson did it with the third year. Just like he did with Nathan. And like with Nathan, he did the most difficult part of the dissection himself. Incarcerated hernias can be treacherous. Don't take it personally. Peterson never lets a first year resident do a hernia repair if it's incarcerated."

CHAPTER 8

CENTRAL LINES

We've gathered on the second floor, ready to begin morning rounds. Barney's in the nurses' station and, as usual, we're sitting there, waiting for him to get off the phone. At last, he hangs up and turns to us.

"That was Peterson. He wants me to help him do a gall bladder that came in through the ER late last night, on a Mrs. Luchetti. Anyone remember her?"

We stand in puzzled silence until Milton speaks up. "Overweight lady, diabetic, gall stones. We saw her in Peterson's outpatient clinic."

"Excellent," Barney says. "You win the prize. You get to scrub with us and pull on a retractor for a thankless hour and a half while we complain that we can't see the operative field. And you, by the way, can't see anything either."

Milton puts on a pained expression, but if he's anything like the rest of us, he's delighted to have the opportunity to scrub on a major case.

"No fooling," Barney says. "We need you to provide exposure."

Then Barney turns to Nathan, and hands him a task list. "You guys have three central lines to put in. Take Philip and get the consents signed. Teach Philip how to put them in, and I'll bet he'll buy you lunch."

Nathan pockets the list, and we make our way quickly through morning rounds, examining each patient, writing orders and notes, discharging a few patients, scribbling a "to-do-list" on our three-by-five cards. It's all the routine activities that we go through whenever we make rounds. When we're finished, Barney and Milton go to the OR to operate on Mrs. Luchetti, while Nathan, Ruth and I set off for the Intensive Care Unit (ICU).

Nathan, Ruth and I arrive in the ICU to see the three patients who require insertion of central lines. According to his chart, Mr. Johansson is a sick, 70 year-old gentleman, on a ventilator. His right kidney was removed for cancer two days ago. He also has a history of cardiac problems, and the urologists are having trouble managing his IV fluids. His remaining kidney is putting out paltry amounts of urine. Twenty-five to thirty milliliters an hour is expected following surgery, but he is making only ten milliliters per hour. The urologists called Dr. Peterson to ask us to place a central line to solve the riddle.

"A central line," Nathan explains, as he scribbles a note in Mr. Johansson's chart, "is just a long IV catheter. We insert them through a large vein beneath the clavicle." He points to a location just below his right collarbone. "There's a really big vein in there, but it's too deep to see under the skin." He looks up at Ruth and me. "Once we get it in, we will thread the catheter all the way into the vena cave, the largest vein in the body. Or, if we can, we may be able to get it to go all the way, into the right atrium of the heart. Then we can use it to assess pressures in the heart. If pressures are low, Mr. Johansson may need more IV fluid. If pressures are high, he may be fluid-overloaded and need diuretics. Or he might require other drugs for his heart. That's for the urologists and cardiologists to figure out."

Ruth nods as she realizes how the various services will be working together. But it all depends on our getting a central line into an elusive vein we can't see.

"I'll show you how to do the first one," Nathan says. "And you can put in the rest."

Nathan takes a sterile kit from the ICU supply closet. It contains a large needle, a very large clear plastic syringe, a guide wire and a long plastic catheter. Before he proceeds, he turns to face me.

"What's the first thing we do?"

"Scrub and sterilize the skin."

"Before that?"

"Put a rolled-up towel under the patient to raise his shoulder to help us hit the subclavian vein?"

"Before that?"

I scratch my head.

"Get a consent form signed and explain the likely complications."

"And what are those complications, Ruth?"

"Infection?" she says with her usual nervous giggle.

"And?" Nathan turns to me.

"Pneumothorax," I say. "We do the procedure blind, so it's possible to hit the pleura and collapse the lung."

"Right. And what's the risk of that happening?"

"Maybe one to three percent?"

"That's a little high, but it's about right. Now, in Mr. Johansson's case we don't have to get the consent signed because the urologists got it from the family." We turn to look at the sleeping, medicated patient. I'm struck by the fact that with all the focus on technical challenges, only Ruth has taken a moment to step aside and look at the patient's face.

"They couldn't get the consent from the patient— he's sedated and full of pain meds. So they got it from his next of kin."

Nathan leads us to Mr. Johansson, and places a rolled-up towel beneath his right chest. "That's to push the subclavian vessels forward." Then Nathan wriggles into a sterile gown, cap and gloves, and drapes the patient so that only the area to be operated on, the upper chest, is exposed. After scrubbing and sterilizing the skin with a disinfectant he injects the skin on the chest wall with Xylocaine, a local anesthetic. "Just like at the dentist," Nathan says with a grin.

I can see that he is chewing gum, and that the speed of his chewing increases as he gets closer to inserting the line.

Nathan then takes the large needle from the sterile kit, attaches the plastic syringe to it, and inserts the needle into the chest just below the left collarbone. He keeps the needle lying parallel to the bone, advancing it slowly toward the opposite shoulder. "I'm staying right on the clavicle," he says. "I can feel the hardness of the bone with the tip of my needle. I don't go deep or I might hit the pleura and collapse the lung."

Nathan is chewing at a furious rate now.

After five or ten seconds of hunting, he penetrates the subclavian vein; this rewards him with a sudden gush of dark red venous blood filling the transparent syringe. "Bingo," he says. He inserts a slender guide-wire through the needle, through the great vein and into the heart. Then he slides a plastic catheter over the guide-wire, advancing it all the way in. We now have a long catheter that extends from the skin all the way into the heart. Nathan connects the catheter to a pressure-measuring device. Then he secures the catheter to the skin with a stitch. Finally, he dresses the wound with disinfectant and gauze.

"What do we do next?" Nathan asks.

"I have no idea," I admit to him. "I've been watching you do the procedure."

"Where's the tip of the catheter?" he asks. "Did we give him a pneumothorax and collapse his lung?"

Finally, I stumble over the answer. "Get a portable chest x-ray!"

"Exactly. And in the meantime?"

I search my memory, but nothing comes to mind.

Nathan takes a stethoscope out of his pocket and lays it on Mr. Johansson's chest. "We play doctor," he says. Nathan is chewing more slowly now. "There is no doubt about it," Nathan says. "There are few sounds in nature as beautiful as normal breath sound. They'd be muffled or absent if we collapsed the lung." He turns to a hovering ICU nurse. "How about we get a portable chest film."

"It's on its way." she says. "Standard procedure after insertion of all central lines."

Then he carefully discards the used drapes and sharp needles into a special red plastic box marked SHARPS. It is full of nasty devices that could easily cut and injure.

"One down," Nathan says as he scribbles a brief procedure note in Mr. Johansson's chart. "Two to go." We move to the next ICU patient who requires a central line. "You put this one in," Nathan says to me. "And I'll help you. The consent form has been signed by the family."

I'm reminded of the surgical truism: see one, do one, teach one. Nathan boasts that he has done more of these procedures in recent months than Dr. Peterson has. And I don't doubt it.

I scan the patient's chart—"Michael Roarty, 35 years old, on a ventilator, motorcycle accident, head trauma, no helmet, major long bone fractures, sepsis." I know I should study the chart, but my eagerness to learn to do this procedure exceeds my obligation to review his medical record. I'm here to learn to do this procedure; I may never see this patient again. I guess I have to admit it: for a surgical resident, the lure of mastering surgical skills is irresistible. They are milestones of skills acquired.

I go through each step I observed when Nathan inserted the line in Mr. Johansson. I placed a rolled towel behind the patient's shoulder, put on a cap, mask and gown, apply the drapes, scrub and disinfect the skin, inject local anesthesia to numb the skin, and penetrate the skin of the chest wall just below the collar bone with the large needle. I do every step. So far, that was not difficult, but now I begin to search for that elusive subclavian vein.

"Not so deep," Nathan warns. "Or you will hit the lung."

I adjust the depth of my needle.

"No!" he shouts as I position the needle incorrectly. "Point the needle toward the opposite shoulder." I try to follow his agitated instructions, but it's difficult to understand precisely what he wants me to do. And the increasing volume of his voice doesn't help any. My anxiety rises in unison, I suspect, with his. Finally, Nathan takes the needle and syringe in his gloved hands and after a few probing movements, hits the vein. The syringe fills with dark red blood. Nathan urges me to remove the syringe and insert the guide wire and long catheter.

"Advance the catheter," he says. "Then stitch it in place to keep it from slipping out."

I am frustrated by my inability to have found the subclavian vein myself, but it is, I remind myself, a blind procedure. Whatever else, I pray I have not given this patient a pneumothorax. I remove the drapes and reach for my stethoscope. Nathan is right—what lovely music breath sounds are.

Finally, we approach the third ICU patient who needs a central line. This is it, I think to myself—pass or fail. I remind myself to review her chart—Mrs. McCall, a 71 year old lady, receiving chemotherapy for metastatic cancer, possible sepsis. But the words roll off me; I really don't care what is written in the chart, as long as it does not say anticoagulation or blood thinners.

She needs a central line for the delivery of medications, but mastering the insertion of a central line is my challenge, not hers. Could she imagine that she is only the second patient in whom I have tried to insert a central line? Of course not. But for every doctor and every procedure, there is a first time. No one begins with their fiftieth procedure. My anxiety rises; I just know I'm going to fail again. I pray I don't give her a pneumothorax. A collapsed lung is the last thing this sick woman needs.

Nathan gowns and gloves with me, and calmly encourages me to go through all the steps of the procedure. He does not harass me or hurry me. I hesitantly advance the needle toward the opposite shoulder. I probe for a moment or two. Nothing. Then, as I change the position of the needle, I am rewarded by gush of dark red venous blood that fills the transparent syringe. Rejoice. I hit the vein! How did I do that? I'm not really sure, but I'll take it. As surgical residents say, I'd rather be lucky than good. I was lucky but I must have learned something from Nathan as well.

"See," Nathan says. "You did fine."

Boy, am I relieved. "Hey, Nathan," I say. "How about some lunch? I'll buy."

"Okay," he says, "But let's listen to her lungs and check her x-rays first."

"Oh yes, of course". How could I have forgotten? Right now, I can leap tall buildings in a single bound. Her breath sounds and X-ray films are normal. We head for the cafeteria. I'm feeling flush that I'm learning new skills.

"By the way," Nathan asks as we stride along. "Suppose we did create a pneumothorax, what would we have done about it?"

We're back to quizzing mode, not even a second for me to savor my triumph.

"Insert a chest tube in the fourth interspace between the ribs and connect the tube to suction." I answer without hesitation, surprised by how easily it comes to me. That's a textbook answer. I read it last night. I've never actually seen a chest tube inserted or removed, and I couldn't imagine doing it myself.

"Philip," Nathan says. "Why don't you read about pneumothorax, and give the students, Barney and me a little lecture about it?"

"A little lecture! Like when?"

"Like this afternoon."

"This afternoon! So soon? Well, there goes my lunch."

While Nathan finishes his second chicken salad sandwich with Barney and the students, I withdraw to a call room where I open the surgery textbook, and read everything I can about pneumothorax. There are volumes and volumes written on the subject, but I scribble the key points on a three-by-five card. At one-thirty, I rejoin our service in the back of the cafeteria, where all of our team sits around an empty cafeteria table. I give my presentation while Milton and Ruth take notes. Barney and Nathan sit back and listen.

"This is it, guys, so sit up and listen. One performance only.

"The lung is held open by surface tension that keeps it stuck to the inner surface of the chest wall. That's good."

Everybody is smiling.

"If the lung collapses, you can't move air in and out to breathe. That's bad. Like a cold, you don't want to have a pneumothorax, and you don't want to give it one to someone else.

"You treat a pneumothorax by inserting a chest tube into the chest cavity in the space between the third and fourth ribs, and you put the tube on suction to keep the lung inflated.

"There is a lot more to talk about, but that's all I had time for."

Milton and Ruth give me a small round of student applause and a big laugh. "Nice job, professor," Ruth says. "You're going to be a great teacher someday."

I thank everyone and note that, as always, I learn more when I teach than when I am a student.

CHAPTER 9

MORBIDITY AND MORTALITY CONFERENCE

At four o'clock, Barney brings our team together, and we walk to the Medical Center amphitheater for M and M Conference. Nathan explains what the conference is all about. "M and M stands for Morbidity and Mortality, Morbidity refers to sickness, and Mortality refers to death. It's a Quality of Care review. Any complication or death that occurs within 30 days of a surgical procedure must be attributed to the procedure, no matter how remote it may seem. It is the most certain way of including and analyzing all complications, and not rationalizing any of them away."

Each surgical service is represented at the conference with a list of all the procedures performed over the past week, and all the complications that occurred with each procedure. Every member of the department of surgery—General Surgery, Plastics, Vascular Surgery—everyone is expected to attend.

"I like this conference," Nathan says. "You learn a lot, and they have good sweet rolls. Forget M and M," He says. "I call it D and D—Death and Doughnuts."

We line up outside the amphitheater door, sign in, grab a cup of coffee and a sweet roll (Nathan takes two), and take a seat. Seating is by no means random. The attending surgeons—Drs. Peterson, Quinn, Raymond,

Benton and others—all sit in the first and second rows. It is as though their gray hair is meant to symbolize wisdom and experience. The residents—Barney, Nathan, myself and all the residents on all the other surgical services—sit in the next three rows. Finally, the medical students fill out the seats in the back of the room. Even though he's currently assigned to the ER, Lenny Goldstein comes to the conference to listen and learn. He nods a greeting and sits down beside me.

Dr. Quinn is a general surgeon who runs this conference. At four-thirty sharp, he rises and walks to the front of the room. "General Surgery II," he calls out in a booming voice. No one is going to snooze through this conference.

The senior resident on the General Surgery Service II, Tony DeMaar, proceeds to the front of the room. DeMaar is short, olive-skinned, in his fifth year of surgical residency. He seems calm enough, even though he's on the hot seat in front of the entire department of surgery. He reads from hand-scribbled notes. "Mr. GT came into the hospital for elective repair of a right inguinal hernia. It was repaired without complications, and he was discharged on the first post-op day. But he returned to the ER the next day with bleeding from the wound. After local exploration in the ER, he was returned to the operating room where the wound was opened widely and re-explored. No specific bleeding vessel was found."

"Was found, not were found," Quinn says, correcting DeMaar's grammar.

"What a shit," Lenny whispers beside me. "Correcting DeMaar's surgical decisions are one thing, but correcting his grammar—that's another matter altogether."

"The wound was thoroughly irrigated and re-closed. Antibiotics were given systemically," DeMaar says.

Before he can continue, Dr. Quinn is on his feet, gruffly interrupting DeMaar. "Tell us about management of the wound. Should it have been opened in the ER or should the patient have been taken directly to the operating room? Was it appropriate to give antibiotics?"

To me, it seems that Quinn's questions are barbed and accusatory, and that he has an answer in mind for each of them. It feels like an inquisition.

"The wound was absolutely dry," DeMaar says. "It was like a desert in there."

"Like a *desert* in there?" Quinn repeats. "What's that supposed to mean?"

A few residents sitting in the middle of the room look up expectantly. "This is no joke," Quinn says glaring at De Maar. "This is the worst decision-making I've ever seen."

The worst decision-making? A bit of exaggeration, I think to myself. This was not exactly a brain transplant.

"When are you going to learn to close an incision in the operating room so it doesn't bleed? You're a fifth year resident!"

DeMaar insists that there was not the slightest hint of bleeding when he closed the fascia and skin at the time of the original operation.

"Well, it bled," Quinn says dryly. "What about his clotting profile? Was he taking aspirin? Heparin? Coumadin?"

"He had been taking Coumadin for a prosthetic aortic valve, but he was off that for three days."

"And his clotting data?"

"His clotting profile and platelet count were all within normal limits, as though he wasn't on any anticoagulation."

"So how do you explain his bleeding?"

"Honestly," DeMaar says. "I don't know. But it wasn't technical. There was no evidence of a bleeding vessel when we opened the wound."

The attendings in the front rows are sitting on the edges of their seats, eager to get into the fray. Before long, the discussion degenerates into a feeding frenzy of opinions with each attending challenging or defending what DeMaar did or did not do.

It sounds like intellectual chaos, but there are good ideas flitting about the room. It also shows that there is a variety of ways to do things. Surgery is an art, and only incompletely a science.

53

The people who examine data for quality assurance purposes compute the number of undesirable events that occur per one hundred cases performed, or per ten thousand cases performed. But in this instance, the underlying issue always is what did we do wrong? What could we do better next time? How do we avoid bleeding next time? It comes down to surgical judgment and technical skill.

"If you were faced with the same situation again," Quinn says to DeMaar. "What would you do differently?"

"I would take him directly to the operating room, and open the wound—that is, if I could get into the OR right away. We couldn't in this case because they were doing an emergency heart."

"What about antibiotics?" Quinn asks.

"We gave intravenous antibiotics."

"Are there any published data to support the use of topical antibiotics to flush a wound."

"There are," DeMaar answers. "And certainly in animal models. But not everyone believes in using them. We did use an antibiotic flush in this patient."

"And how did the patient do?"

"Fine. We saw him in clinic after five days at home. There was no evidence of further bleeding."

"Well, at least someone on your service knows how to close a wound." Quinn says.

"Anything to add?" he asks turning to Dr. Raymond, the attending on the case.

"No, that about covers it."

DeMaar sits down with a nervous grin; he endured another of Quinn's diatribes, and lived to tell the tale.

Dr. Quinn then calls on our service. "General Surgery I."

Barney stands up and walks to the front of the room to describe our patient, Mr. Hall, the patient who died of the ruptured four-centimeter aortic aneurysm. Before Barney can finish his presentation, Dr. Quinn is on his feet riddling him with questions.

"Why didn't you simply assume that the aneurysm was the cause of his discomfort? You didn't need another diagnosis."

Barney buttons his coat as though he were wearing a bulletproof vest.

"He had a palpable impulse on physical examination," Barney says, "suggestive of a hernia."

Quinn nods his head. "He had a known aneurysm that could account for his symptoms. He didn't need a second diagnosis."

Lenny Goldstein sits back with a self-satisfied smile. That was his position all along.

But not all the attendings in the front row agree, and their heated discussion degenerates into statements and restatements of each attending's opinion. After several minutes of persistent wrangling, Dr. Quinn asks Dr. Benton, Chief of Vascular Surgery, to comment on the risks of rupture of a four-centimeter aneurysm.

Benton rises and scans those present in the room, his steel gray eyes sweep across the audience of attendings and residents. I often heard residents describe Benton as surgically skilled and imperturbable.

"We really don't know the risks of not operating and just observing an aneurysm that small," Benton says. "I don't know of any data in the vascular surgery literature to guide us."

Dr. Quinn digests that for a few moments.

Dr. Peterson then stands to summarize what we found on physical examination—signs and symptoms consistent with an inguinal hernia. I think he's protecting Benton, or perhaps himself. After several minutes of inconclusive wrangling, Quinn asks Barney his usual wrap up question; "Knowing what you know now, what would you have done differently."

Barney looks directly at Quinn. He knows he has Benton and Peterson on his side. "Sir," he says. "I probably would do just what we did in this case, but I'd try to get an answer about a possible hernia that first evening, not the following day. Even so, we can't just operate on everybody who walks in the door with a small aneurysm without taking some surgical risk. Aneurysms carry a small but undeniable risk of mortality."

Quinn ponders that argument for a moment. "Good point," he says finally.

I find the interchange between the attendings and residents fascinating; at least I do as long as I am just observing the battlefield and I am not caught up in the middle of it. Thank God we did not give any of the patients a pneumothorax today when we inserted the central lines, or it might be Barney or me up there in the hot seat.

I know that this conference is supposed to educate the residents, and grilling us is one way to do that. We're all a little wiser, learning from each other's mistakes.

M and M is all part of the educational process to make us think of the consequences of our surgical decisions. I finally realize that, that is why the residents are called upon to defend the actions taken, rather than the attending defending their decisions. It is practice for legal sparring and for the oral portion of the final examination for General Surgery. Still, there are moments when I am listening to Quinn and I can't help but wonder what he's really like. Can you imagine being a child and having him as a father? I'd rather not think about it.

CHAPTER 10

LAST DAY ON GENERAL SURGERY

This is my last day on General Surgery. We finished evening rounds, and we are free to leave. But somehow I feel a twinge of conscience leaving the patients under the care of a resident on night call who doesn't know the first thing about them.

But those introspective feelings don't last more than a moment or two. I'm not on call, and I have no outstanding charts waiting to be dictated. As soon as I can get the gumption, I am going to do battle with the traffic on this rainy night and drive home to have dinner with my wife and children.

Outside, the city lights are just coming on. I head down to the university cafeteria to buy a cup of coffee. I find an available table where I am joined by a couple of medical students who are between rotations; they pepper me with questions. After a few minutes, Nathan strolls into the cafeteria to sit with us as well. Knowing him, I suspect that he will eat dinner in the cafeteria, then go home to have dinner with his wife.

"What's it like being a first year resident?" one of the students asks me.

"Do you actually get to do anything or do you just have to do scut work like we're doing now?" asks another.

"Oh, no," I tell them, "I just completed three months on Dr. Peterson's General Surgery service and, to tell you the truth, I learned much more than I ever expected—skills and judgment that will apply to many areas of surgery."

"Like what? Were you there for any cardiac arrests?"

"No," I say, sipping my coffee. "Dr. Peterson says that he does not permit his patients to have cardiac arrests."

Everyone laughs.

"It's been a great experience. During the three months, I operated on five hernias, first assisted on one elective tracheotomy, did three lymph node biopsies and removed a number of breast lesions. The tracheotomy was more difficult than I expected with a lot of bleeding. As you can imagine, bleeding in the neck can be dangerous. I also did a number of minor superficial procedures including excision of simple cysts and small lipomas from the skin. It's not big-time surgery, but Hey! A guy has to start somewhere—right?" The medical students appear to hang on my every word, so I continue.

"I've learned to recognize the difference between benign and malignant skin lesions, just by looking at them. Basal cell carcinoma is a relatively benign lesion that spreads by local invasion. Squamous cell carcinoma is more aggressive, it spreads by the lymphatic channels. Melanoma is the most aggressive. It grows and spreads any which way it wants to, and it can be lethal. But the most important thing I learned was pre-op and post-op care." I stop talking long enough to take another sip of coffee.

Since all eyes are still fixed on me I keep going.

"I was especially pleased that I learned to put in central lines. One of the most useful things I learned was how to use forceps and scissors when dissecting tissue. I'm sure those skills are going to be useful whatever field of surgery I pursue."

"I'm interested in Pathology," a female medical student says. "But I'm not sure. Did you get a chance to go to the Pathology Lab and look at the excised tissues with the pathologists? Did you learn anything?"

"Yes," I assure her.

"I always found it to be quite informative. There is a truism in medicine that goes like this:

"Internists know everything, but do nothing.

"Surgeons do everything, but know nothing.

"Psychiatrists know nothing and do nothing.

"Pathologists (the doctors who do the autopsies) know everything, but a day too late."

CHAPTER 11

NEUROSURGERY

Today is my first day on the Neurosurgical service. Our senior resident is the unflappable Andy Kovalchik, a mature, circumspect man who is beginning his required seventh year of Neurosurgical residency. With all the education and experience he has accumulated, he is just a few hurdles away from being an attending neurosurgeon himself.

I am the only junior resident on the neurosurgical team, although we do have two eager medical students, Eric and Estelle. As we make rounds, Andy always takes the time to introduce us to the patients as though we were important in the diagnostic and therapeutic hierarchy. We inspect and document the condition of the patient's scalp, skull and back incisions, depending on what surgery had been performed. Andy also assigns us responsibilities for checking lab values and x-ray reports. We send two patients home, and meet two new admissions; both are here for back surgery to remove protruding lumbar discs. My three-by-five note cards are back in action, covered front and back with scribbles, tasks and new information. What would I do without them?

"A couple of times a week," Andy tells us, "one of the attending neurosurgeons will make rounds with us.

But there are no attendings with us this morning because they have all been summoned to an early morning meeting with the dean of the medical school."

Our rounds take us from one patient to another until finally we meet Mrs. Hanson, a lady who is scheduled for brain surgery this morning. She is a sad-looking, fifty-two year old lady with a recently diagnosed brain tumor.

"We have treated her with steroids for the past several days," Andy tells us, "to reduce brain swelling."

"The headache is a little better," she says. "And I haven't had any seizures since you put me on that new medicine. But I haven't slept either. I need some rest," she says with a sniffle. At last, she begins to weep.

And who can blame her? She is just minutes away from undergoing surgery on her brain, a procedure that is bound to leave some residual untoward effect.

"I'm sorry," Andy says, resting his hand on her shoulder. He seems moved by her tears. "Today is your operation. Afterward, we'll see if we can't give you something for sleep."

When we leave Mrs. Hanson's room, we stop in the hall where Andy lowers his voice, and speaks to the students and myself.

"This patient has what looks on x-ray to be a glioblastoma. It is one of the most common types of brain tumors and also one of the most resistant to treatment." He puts his hands together; finger tip to finger tip, then spreads his fingers into what loosely approximates a cube. "The skull acts like a rigid box," he says. "As the tumor grows, it is limited by the skull, and this raises the pressure in the skull and the cerebrospinal fluid in the brain. It is this increased pressure that causes patients with brain tumors to have headaches and seizures."

Then he explains the neurosurgeon's therapeutic strategy, "We're giving Mrs. Hanson steroids and mannitol because they lower the pressure in the skull, at least temporarily. Unfortunately, in some patients, insomnia is a substantial side-effect of the steroids."

"What is the prognosis?" Estelle asks Andy.

"Poor, very poor. The tumor is incurable, but it still dictates our strategy. We remove as much of the tumor as we can to reduce pressure in the skull, and give the tumor room to expand."

As I think about it, I am struck by the horror of it all—a mass of tumor cells reproducing without restraint inside this lady's skull. It is like weeds growing in her favorite flower pot.

"Does she know about the tumor?" Estelle asks.

"Oh, yes," Andy says. "Heineken is her attending. He explains everything to all his patients. I know he talked to her about the tumor and our treatment strategy because I was there when he spoke to her."

"It's so bizarre," Estelle, says. "With all this serious disease, Mrs. Hanson seems to be concerned only about sleeping."

"Yes," Andy says. "It is interesting how different people react to bad health news. Some people simply deny it. Others wring their hands and obsess about it. Still others focus on a distraction—like a lack of sleep. I think that's what she's doing, but I'm not sure. He stares off for a moment. "I don't know how I'd react to a hopeless diagnosis, but I'm sure I would appreciate a good night's sleep that would provide at least some temporary distraction and relief from the worry. Can you imagine what it is like for her? The moment she awakens, the first thought that comes to her is about her incurable illness." Andy nods his head. If only his kindness could help her.

Andy continues his introspection. "It used to be that families would ask doctors and nurses to withhold information from their patients. That was quite common in the 1950's and 1960's. And the doctors would go along with it in order to spare patients relentless anxiety. But nowadays, that's all changed. We speak openly with patients, giving them time for getting their affairs in order. And that is how it should be. Our contract as caregivers is primarily with the patients, and only incidentally with the family."

Returning to Mrs. Hanson, Estelle asks, "Would chemo help her?"

"I'm afraid not." Andy says. "Not a tumor with this histology. Often, radiation will shrink a tumor, or slow it down, just temporarily. It may buy time, maybe six months to a year."

Six months to a year; it doesn't sound like much, but it's precious, especially of it's the last year of a person's life. I must admit that I never thought of life expectancy in such concrete terms before.

We finish rounds at seven-fifteen, and walk as a group to the operating room. On the way, we encounter Dr. Heineken, the Chief of Neurosurgery, Mrs. Hanson's attending neurosurgeon. He's an enormous man—six feet two or three, two hundred seventy-five pounds, maybe more. His moon face is topped by an incongruous bristly blond crew cut. He does not wear the usual hospital lab coat or green scrubs that everyone else does; instead, for reasons known only to him, he wears his own all-white scrubs and a white lab coat. This morning, on our way to the operating room, he rushes past us, going in the opposite direction murmuring that he forgot something in his office. He is a startling figure, his lab coat flapping like a great white fluke; a surgical Moby Dick.

In the operating room, Dr. Heineken and Andy gently take Mrs. Hanson's hands, comforting her as she slips under the beneficent spell of anesthesia. Sleep, at last, for this anxious, sleep-starved woman. When she is asleep, the anesthesiologist inserts a breathing tube in her airway. I watch him adjust its position. He must be certain that the tube is not kinked, and that it is connected securely to the anesthesia apparatus and to the patient.

When Mrs. Hanson is anesthetized, Andy puts her angiogram on the illuminated view box on the operating room wall. This shows the blood vessels that supply the brain. A cutoff is readily apparent where the tumor has intruded, blocking the flow of blood. We cannot see the tumor itself. What we see is the absence of the cerebral circulation where it is impeded by the presence of the tumor.

"These indirect images of tumors are going to be replaced by more direct ones," Andy says. "There are new devices called Scans that are not far off for clinical use. I've seen the images and they are unbelievable. Even though the tissue density of the tumor is similar to the normal brain, you can actually see the tumor!"

Dr. Heineken, Andy and I withdraw to the scrub sink outside the operating room. After scrubbing our hands and forearms for five minutes, we re-enter the operating room, and gown and glove for surgery. Dr. Heineken directs me to stand between Mrs. Hanson and a masked, gowned scrub nurse named Lois.

"I scrub on all the neurosurgical cases," Lois says with pride. She speaks with a shrill, squeaky voice. "It's my specialty. I even come in on the weekends for emergencies, if I happen to be in town." She laughs a soprano laugh.

The operating room is set up differently for neurosurgery than it is for general surgery in that we have not one, but two, large instrument tables. They're about four feet long, set at angles to one another, and are arranged in two tiers with one table higher than the other. I feel like I'm standing on the field at a baseball game with the stands rising up around me. Both tables are laid out with twenty-five or thirty sterilized instruments. I've never seen most of these devices before because they are designed specifically for use in Neurosurgery.

Another difference from General Surgery concerns the position of the patient. Mrs. Hanson is not lying on her back as the patients are when we repair their hernias or perform abdominal surgery. Instead, she is propped up, like someone sitting up in bed, reading a magazine. All except the upper part of her head is covered with sterile drapes, similar to the way a barber covers a man's neck and shoulders when he is about to provide a haircut. The Operating Room nurses shaved her head, in her room, in preparation for today's surgery. Poor woman, I think. I'll bet that a shaved head posed another emotional stress for her. Sadly, we have left her with little of her feminine pride.

Dr. Heineken and Andy begin the procedure. They take seats on tall bar-room-style stools, one on each side of Mrs. Hanson.

We begin. Andy makes a silver dollar-size circular incision in Mrs. Hanson's scalp at a location that should place him directly over the tumor. He leaves about a third of the circle uncut to provide blood supply for healing after the surgery. This leaves a man hole cover of scalp that will act as a hinged flap. Andy temporarily folds the scalp flap back, and then drills half a dozen small holes in the skull in the form of a circle.

Finally, he uses a pneumatically-driven saw to join the drilled holes. This permits him to remove the silver dollar disc of skull bone. The tile walls of the operating room rings with the staccato rap of a pneumatic drill and saw; these are such coarse carpenter's tools used to provide access to the delicate, protected brain.

For one moment, I am struck by how much the outer surface of the brain resembles that of a cauliflower.

Now that the brain is exposed, Andy and Dr. Heineken carefully separate the folds of the brain with spatulas, flat stainless steel instruments that are as smooth and shiny as polished butter knives. The brilliant overhead lights reflect erratically off these stainless-steel instruments as Dr. Heineken manipulates the spatulas to expose the tumor.

The brain is pale gray, and divided into segments. The tumor mass lies deep at the base of one or more of these segments. Once he has identified the location of the tumor, Dr. Heineken inserts a catheter into the mass to suck out as much tumor as possible.

"Glioblastomas have microscopic tentacles," he says. "And they insinuate themselves among and around the normal brain tissue. It would be impossible to completely remove all the tentacles without removing so much brain that we would cripple this patient." He looks up at the medical students. "Our intent here is not to completely excise the tumor—it can't be done. All we can hope for is that we provide sufficient space for the tumor to grow without imposing pressure on the remaining healthy brain—at least for a while."

I can't help but reflect on what a primitive state of science this is. It seems barbaric to be dissecting someone's brain just to provide space for an unwanted tumor to grow. But currently, that is all we have. Surgery is but a graceful capitulation.

I watch Dr. Heineken's meaty hands manipulate the spatulas and the suction catheter. He moves with uncanny grace, without the slightest tremor. I've heard him say that he drinks no caffeine, tea, or alcohol, and that he does not smoke.

For twenty minutes, Andy and Dr. Heineken draw out tumor cells and meticulously remove small formless fragments of gray tissue. When we excise all the tumor mass that we can, and bleeding has been controlled, the disc of skull (the silver dollar) that was removed is returned to its rightful place and wired back into place.

The surgeons bandage Mrs. Hanson's head, the anesthesiologist reverses anesthesia and they transfer her out of the operating room and into the Recovery Room. When she is fully awake and breathing on her own, the Recovery Room nurses transfer her from the Recovery Room to the Neurosurgical Intensive Care Unit.

We join Mrs. Hanson and her husband in the ICU. She is able to speak, but her words are garbled with residual anesthesia. As expected after surgery, she complains of pain in her scalp and skull. Ironically, the brain itself—the recipient of all the sensory neurons and pain receptors in the entire body—feels no pain.

***

We start rounds in the ICU at six-thirty in the morning. Mrs. Hanson is doing remarkably well on her first post-op day, Andy points out that she has some motor weakness, probably from all the manipulation of her brain. And hopefully, most of her weakness will be temporary. "She is awake and alert, and speaking, if somewhat confused." But Andy is pleased. She is still on steroids and probably will remain so for a long time, perhaps the rest of her life. As soon as she is able, Andy will get her up and about, and into physical therapy. And, as promised, he will give her something for sleep.

***

Today we have one scheduled case, Mrs. Willibrand, a seventy-year old lady who has brain metasases from a primary breast cancer. Evidently, before the primary tumor in her breast was removed, it sent off clusters of cells, some of which took hold in her brain. When we walk into her room, we find her sitting bolt upright in bed, her head shaved, an IV in a vein in her arm. She grips her husband's arm fiercely while they wait for a Transportation orderly to take her to the operating room. "When Dr. Peterson operated on my breast," Mrs. Willibrand says, "he told me he thought he got it all. But now this. And what if it becomes infected?"

"Now, Mrs. Willibrand", Andy says. "Infections after brain surgery are not very common."

She stares off into space, apparently unmoved by Andy's minimal assurances.

I suspect that the reason she has focused on a fear of infection is to avoid thinking about the greater problem—a cancer is growing in her brain!

She grips her husband's arm so tightly that when she releases it, I can see his skin blanched white from where her five fingers had gripped him. She looks terrified, and who can blame her? An operation on her brain! I would like to encourage her with some kind words, but nothing I could say would be helpful. In truth, I would be as frightened as she is if I were in her position. I try not to think about it.

After we leave her room, Andy tells us that our approach to this lesion will be different than what it was for Mrs. Hanson. "We will open and close the skull in the same way we did in Mrs. Hanson," he says. "But in Mrs. Willibrand, we will try to remove the entire tumor, intact, without spilling any of the malignant cells. Unlike the diffuse tentacles of a glioblastoma in Mrs. Hanson, this tumor metastasis should be discrete, firm and nodular, and we'll try to remove it in its entirety"

On the way to the operating room, Andy introduces me to the attending surgeon for Mrs. Willibrand's case. He is Dr. Albert Randazzo, a lean, dark-haired man with a relaxed easy way about him and a constant ironic smile.

"I had a meeting with the dean yesterday," he says to Andy as we stride along. "He wants us to take more medical students on our service. I told him yes. Then he asked us to think about providing more services for the medical school—an extra teaching clinic, possibly an off-site clinic. Again, I said yes. I kept saying yes, yes, yes— and he kept asking for more, more, more. I'll tell you; that man won't take yes for an answer."

I listen carefully as we walk, for I never knew about all the political maneuvering that goes on behind the scenes in a university medical center. As a medical student, it has always been outside my realm to know about the push and pull of all these internal strains and the competition for resources.

Dr. Randazzo, Andy and I head to the locker room where we change into clean scrubs. Then we scrub our hands and forearms, enter the operating room, gown and glove. We stand beside the draped, anesthetized Mrs. Willibrand. Dr. Randazzo and Andy discuss precisely where they want to make the scalp incision. Once it's settled, our scrub nurse, Lois, hands Andy a scalpel and skin clips, then other instruments as he requires them in unbroken rapid-fire sequence. She anticipates what instrument he needs. Yesterday, I was so uncertain about my role and responsibilities that I didn't notice the seamless relationship between Lois and the surgeons. But now I can see it clearly; a well-choreographed, a pas de deux for surgeon and nurse. I also can see why surgeons want their own cadre of specialized nurses to work with them, day in and day out. Unfortunately that seldom is possible.

Andy carefully makes a semi-circular incision in the scalp, and applies metal clips to the cut edges of the wound to control bleeding. Then he drills and opens the skull, just as he did yesterday. I look down into the wound as Andy and Dr. Randazzo probe deeply between the convoluted folds of the brain. They are searching for the clusters of malignant cells.

"There it is," Dr. Randazzo says. The circulating nurse rolls the dissecting microscopes into place. The room is silent except for the rhythmic hiss of the anesthesia machine breathing for Mrs. Willibrand.

Suddenly, without warning, the intense concentration in the room is broken by a rasping, buzzing sound as a fat iridescent green fly sweeps over the exposed brain.

"Shit!" Dr. Randazzo yells. "Cover the brain!"

Andy waves the fly away with a sterile towel, while Lois scrambles to place a sterile towel over Mrs. Willibrand's exposed brain.

"Sterile fly swatter," Randazzo says whimsically. He reaches out as though he were expecting a surgical instrument to be slapped in his palm. The circulating nurse runs out of the room to return with a fist-full of colored plastic fly swatters. She hands one to Dr. Randazzo.

"Blue," he growls. "My favorite color fly swatter. Perfect for the operating room."

Andy and I watch as a great contest unfolds: Dr. Randazzo versus the Fly. The fly buzzes back and forth, back and forth, relentless energy in motion.

"It's the caffeine." Dr. Randazzo says dryly. "Too much time spent buzzing around the coffee pot."

Andy and I wave our sterile towels over the anesthetized Mrs. Willibrand. At the same time, Lois covers the exposed brain with a sterile towel, and keeps the pest away from her instruments. Then the room again falls silent. Where is that fly? It's somewhere in the room, but where? All I can hear is the regular wheezing pulse of the anesthesia machine.

"There"—Lois squeaks, pointing to the opposite wall.

"Where?" Randazzo asks.

"Over there. On the wall."

Andy and Randazzo chase the pest while Lois and I try to protect Mrs. Willibrand and exposed instruments. We swat and chase, but the pest lands and contaminates first one tray of 30 surgical instruments, and then the others. Then it contaminates the sterile drape that covers Mrs. Willibrand's head, but fortunately, does not contaminate her brain.

"No-o-o," Lois squeals, guarding her instruments. At last, Dr. Randazzo catches up with the pest. He flattens it with one decisive swat, then drops to his knees, pounding it to two dimensions—length and width with no height.

Dr. Randazzo emerges the victor. He stands with his hands on his hips, laughing at the absurdity of the situation—a common housefly in our most sacred space. The circulating nurse arrives with a Kleenex to carry away the mashed   corpse. Then, each of us takes our turn changing our gowns and scrubbing once again. One by one, soiled contaminated surgical instruments, towels and drapes are exchanged for clean ones.

All the while, the patient sleeps, oblivious of the drama that has just taken place above her. Of course, Andy will document the great contest in his operative report, and, unless I am very much mistaken, everyone working in the operating room suite already knows about our adventure. Bizarre episodes such as these do not go unreported. For a moment, I think of Mrs. Willibrand's obsession with fear of infection.

After we've all re-scrubbed, we return to Mrs. Willibrand. The room suddenly seems eerily quiet as we return to normal pace of the operation. Fortunately, the entire tumor can be removed, and after thirty minutes,

Andy and Dr. Randazzo have it out. We send it to Pathology where the pathologist can examine it while we wait. After a few minutes, a disembodied voice speaks to us through the intercom speaker on the wall. It is Bruno, our surgical pathologist.

"You have clear margins," he says. "Free of tumor all around."

"Wonderful!" Andy exclaims. That is what we have been striving for.

***

In the hall, outside the ICU, we meet Mr. Willibrand who has been waiting to hear about his wife.

"How is she doing, doctor?" he asks with a deeply furrowed look.

"She's doing fine," Dr. Randazzo says. "You'll be able to see her in a few minutes, but she won't be really awake for another couple of hours."

"Were you able to get all the tumor out?"

"Yes, I think so. But as you know, we can't always be sure about these things."

"Yes, of course, and how did the operation go?"

"Just fine." Dr. Randazzo says, "But, there is something I should tell you..."

It is at this point that I decide to stretch my legs and take a little walk

CHAPTER 12

NEUROSURGERY CONSULTS

Andy, the medical students and I begin morning rounds. We have one new patient, Lawrence Minor, a burly 27 year-old man who works on the loading dock at the local post office. He is Dr. Randazzo's patient, and has been undergoing diagnostic tests for persistent lower back pain.

Mr. Minor lies quietly on his bed when we meet him. "My back," he says. "It's not bad when I lie down, but it's unbearable when I'm standing up."

"The pain," Andy asks. "Does it radiate anywhere, or does it stay in your lower back?"

"It goes to the back of my leg. On the right."

Andy raises Mr. Minor's left leg, his uninvolved limb, keeping it straight at the knee. Straight left leg raising elicits wincing and a little guarding, but when Andy performs the same maneuver on the right, his symptomatic leg, Mr. Minor writhes and howls in pain, his voice carrying out into the corridor. Reflexively, he shoves Andy roughly away. "Sorry, doc," he says with an embarrassed look.

Andy turns to address the medical students and me.

"Mr. Minor," he says, "Has the classic symptoms of a protruding lumbar disc. His symptoms are textbook.

I've seen his myelogram. The x-rays show a lumbar disc protruding out and pressing on the sciatic nerve. That's what's causing all the pain. It's pressure on the nerve. But the patient feels it as though the pain originated from somewhere down in his leg, the area supplied by the nerve."

The medical students nod silently. I suspect that each of them is promising him or herself to review the anatomy as soon as they have the opportunity to do so. I know because I am promising the same thing to myself.

Andy turns back to Mr. Minor. "Transportation should be here any minute, Mr. Minor. They'll take you to the operating room, and Dr. Randazzo and I will meet you there." While he's speaking, Andy goes through Mr. Minor's chart, checking to be certain that all the paperwork is complete for surgery. As we leave his room, he gives Mr. Minor a thumbs up, and we head to the operating room.

On the way we encounter Lenny Goldstein walking in the opposite direction. He tells me he's on Dr. Peterson's service now, and that the two of them are getting along famously. I wish I were a fly on the wall, witnessing the two of them showing off, like a pair of dueling medical encyclopedias. I'll bet Peterson has never had a resident who was so overflowing with clinical knowledge.

Dr. Randazzo, Andy, the students and I join Mr. Minor in the operating room. Mr. Minor has been given general anesthesia, a tube has been inserted in his airway to secure his ventilation, and we carefully roll him over onto his stomach on the operating table. Now that the airway is secure, Andy and Dr. Randazzo can feel comfortable operating on Mr. Minor while he is lying on his stomach. After he's been turned over, the anesthesiologist checks and rechecks the position of the tube in his airway.

Several days ago, Mr. Minor had a myelogram, an x-ray where contrast material was injected into his spinal canal to visualize the vertebrae and discs of his lower back. Andy puts Mr. Minor's x-ray films up on the illuminated view box on the operating room wall. It demonstrates that some of the discs in his back are compressing the roots of one of his lumbar nerves. This causes the referred pain. The surgeon's task is to perform a procedure which will take the pressure off the nerve.

Dr. Randazzo, Andy and I scrub, gown and glove. The medical students stand off to the side, observing what they can from a distance. It is difficult to see in the small opening through which surgeons are operating. Dr. Randazzo and Andy do the case while I stand beside the patient, gently pulling on a retractor to provide the surgeons with exposure so they can see where to operate. The surgeons make slow and cautious progress.

I hold a retractor where they put me to give them exposure, but I'm no more than a blind robot. It's not gratifying, but I'm not complaining. I'm here to help as well as learn.

After sixty minutes, they finish the case and close the wound. We turn Mr. Minor onto his back and the anesthesiologist turns off the anesthesia. When he is demonstrably awake, we slide Mr. Minor onto a gurney and wheel him into the Recovery Room. Andy writes post-op orders, and then he invites me to accompany him to see some consults.

As we walk to see the first patient, he shows me a Consult Request Sheet, a salmon-colored handwritten form which acts as an official communication between physicians:

Patient: Jacob Swift. Fifty-one year old white male, recent onset of headaches and seizures...

He snatches the sheet away before I can read any more, then takes on the air of a scientific examiner. "What's the first diagnosis you think of in a case like this—headaches and recent onset of seizures in a fifty-one year old man?"

"A brain tumor?"

"Are you asking me or telling me?"

PHILIP B. DOBRIN, M.D.

Before I can answer, he asks. "What's the first diagnostic test you want to order?"

I'm thinking. . .

"You said a tumor," he prompts. "What kind of tumor?"

"A glioblastoma, like Mrs. Hanson?"

"Could be. Or?"

"A metastasis, spread from a tumor that started elsewhere."

"And what's the mnemonic for tumors that originate elsewhere but metastasize to the brain?"

"P T Barnum Loves My Kids—Pharynx, Testis, Breast, Lung, Melanoma, Kidney."

"And of all those tumors, which are most common?"

"Breast and lung?"

"And in a male?"

"Lung."

"Right."

This is gratifying. I'm thinking as fast as Andy wants me to think.

"And at what age are most lung cancers diagnosed?"

"Uh... early fifties?"

"Mr. Swift smokes and is fifty-one. So, before you start ordering exotic tests for a possible brain tumor, what routine test would you like to see?"

"A chest x-ray?"

Andy gives me a thumbs up. "Let's go to X-ray."

"There is a lot of wisdom in medicine," He says as we descend the stairs. "And here is a typical example. When searching for a diagnosis; "Look for horses, not for zebras; look for the commonplace, not the obscure."

In the X-ray department, we ask several of the radiologists to examine Mr. Swift's chest films with us. Each of them agrees to do so but at the moment, they all are occupied reading films. However, Dr. Vasquez, the chief of the Radiology Department, agrees to review the films with us. He is the quintessential diagnostician, legendary in his ability to identify and predict loosely

76

associated diagnoses. Vasquez attended an Ivy League school, and it has been said that no one at University Medical Center has ever seen him not wearing his beloved Ivy League striped tie. He must have a barrel-full of them. More importantly, no one at University Medical Center ever remembers him missing a routine diagnosis, the more obscure the better.

Dr. Vasquez comes strutting out of his cubicle with a cocky, rocking motion, a matador eager to face the bull. He seats himself in front of a large x-ray view box plastered with films, and puts up Mr. Swift's films.

"In recent years, I've become specialized as a neuroradiologist. Just brain and spinal cord, so I don't often get to read plain old chest x-rays anymore. So," he says taking a deep breath, "let's see what I can do."

A little self-deprecation, I think to myself. All part of the Vasquez image.

Vasquez puts up Mr. Swift's chest x-rays and the three of us squint at the gray and black shadows, abstracts of Mr. Swift's heart and lungs, ribs and spine. Most of what we see looks normal.

"But there's something suspicious there." Vasquez points to a subtle mass in the left upper lobe of the lung.

"There's trouble," Vasquez says. "Looks like a tumor to me." He takes a moment to examine a lateral view of the chest, and then nods his head dolefully. "It's a tumor. You can bet on it."

Unfortunately, such an opinion from Vasquez is about as discouraging as a comparable report from a pathologist. We thank him and head back upstairs to see the patient.

***

Mr. Swift is a slight man, sitting passively in bed, watching television. He is alone, his room dimmed by drawn window shades. He wears a solemn look with dark circles under his eyes, and exhibits the hoarse, phlegm-rattled voice of a chronic smoker. The second and third fingers of his right hand are yellow with permanent tobacco stains. We introduce ourselves and ask him about his medical history—how long he's had headaches and seizures, any history of head trauma, and what medications he's taking.

He turns down the television sound, but leaves the picture on, a soap opera about young doctors and nurses working in a hospital. He continues to watch it with occasional glances, even while he's talking with us, real doctors standing in front of him. In fact, he seems more interested in the fictional story on the television screen than he is in us or his own real illness.

"The seizures started a week or so ago," he says. "But I've had headaches for weeks. Aspirin doesn't touch them." He snatches a quick glance now and then at the TV screen.

"How much do you smoke?" Andy asks.

"About two packs a day," Mr. Swift says between furtive glances at the television screen.

"For how long?"

"Since I was twelve."

Two packs a day for forty years. That would be an assault on anyone's lungs.

I listen to his lungs, pressing my stethoscope against his back. But he coughs incessantly, and it's difficult to hear his breath sounds. It is exasperating. "Open your mouth," I say impatiently, "and take a big breath. In and out . . . "

He complies.

As I lean forward to listen to his heart, I see a package of unfiltered Camel cigarettes and a Bic cigarette lighter bulging in his left breast pocket. They are his personal property, undeniably convenient, aimed like a dagger at his heart.

When we leave Mr. Swift, Andy reviews the surgical strategy he is contemplating. "If a person suddenly develops a seizure or complains of a persistent headache—and there's no history of head trauma—think brain tumor.

"Mr. Swift needs a work-up. If he's got a single metastasis in his brain and we think we can get it out, we'll go for it. But if there is more than one metastasis, we won't pursue them. There are probably more that we can't see yet, and taking out multiple lesions would be crippling. It would destroy too much brain."

Andy writes his impressions and recommendations in Mr. Swift's chart. They raise a lot of questions. Where else might he have metastases beside the brain? In other locations in his lung? In his liver? Can the tumor in his lung be removed by thoracic surgery? His physicians will have to get the oncologists and radiation therapists involved.

"I suspect we won't be seeing Mr. Swift again," Andy says. "But Radiation Oncology will."

"How much time do you think he has?" I ask.

Andy shrugs. "It's hard to say. But if I were him, I wouldn't start reading War and Peace or buying long-playing records."

It's irreverent, but it's the kind of remark residents say to sound clever, and to keep from identifying too closely with hopelessly ill patients. As we leave, I can't dispel the image of those cigarettes and the BIC lighter in his breast pocket. As a medical student, smokers always brushed me off when I counseled them about the hazards of smoking.

"Hey, doc," they would say with breezy self-confidence. "You've got to die of something."

That's what they say; if only they knew and what misery awaits them.

"We have one more consult," Andy says. "Something different. Do you know Mike O'Brien, the senior resident on Neurology?"

"I've heard his name…"

"He's a real character. He called me about a 'sidewalk consult,' something unofficial that he thought we might find interesting." Andy pages O'Brien, and the three of us meet in the hall on the third floor.

Mike O'Brien is a short, pale-skinned resident with flaming red hair. One corner of his mouth chronically droops, giving him an expression of perpetual disdain. He overflows with intellectual energy, speaking in short choppy sentences with just a hint of Irish brogue, while he bobs up and down on the balls of his feet. "I've got this Mrs. Woodson," he says. "She's the wife of the mayor of Springdale." He points vaguely to the west. "As you can imagine, in that little burg, Mr. Mayor gets all the attention—the newspaper, television, even their once-a-week throw-a-way paper full of used cars and pizza ads."

O'Brien puts his hands in his pants pocket and jingles loose change. "Last week, Mrs. Woodson started having seizures. I actually saw her have one. It looked like a grand mal to me." He turns to me. "You know, tonic extension of the arms and legs, then jerky clonic movements." He gives us a demonstration in the hall while visitors and patients passing by stop and stare at the show. "But there's something funny about them," he says. "Her arm movements are all on one side. They should be bilateral. Not only that," he says. "When she has a seizure, she never bites her tongue or strikes her head or collides with anything or anybody. Also, her EEG looks pretty normal."

O'Brien puts his hands on his hips, and juts out his jaw. "You know what I think? You want to know? I think they're factitious—fake seizures to get our attention so ol' Mr. Mayor doesn't get all the limelight."

"I've read about factitious seizures," I say. "But I never thought I'd see one."

"Me neither," O'Brien says. "But I've got a plan, and I want you guys to be my witnesses."

Andy agrees, and the three of us walk down the hall to Mrs. Woodson's private room.

Mrs. Woodson lies in bed watching television, a fifty year old gray-haired lady without makeup, inundated by well-wishers' flowers and extravagant gift baskets.

"Mrs. Woodson," O'Brien says, "These doctors are here to help us diagnose your seizures."

Mrs. Woodson's eyes light up when she learns she'll be the center of attention. Andy and I wait at the doorway, just inside the room, while O'Brien walks around to behind the headboard of Mrs. Woodson's bed. He lowers the electric bed so she's lying flat. Then he slips his hand beneath her neck.

"Mrs. Woodson has seizures," he says with the air of a grand professor. "We'd like to study them while they're happening, but we never know exactly when that will be. Fortunately, there is something we can do." O'Brien presses his fingers lightly against the back of Mrs. Woodson's neck. "Right here, in the back of the neck, all the nerves go from the brain down to the body. Most of the nerves are protected by the bony spine," he says, pressing lightly on her spine. "But in some people, there's one great big nerve that runs separate from the spinal column, the Main Nerve. Pressure on the Main Nerve will cause some people to have seizures."

This is nuts, I think to myself. There's no such thing as the Main Nerve. Or maybe I fell asleep during Neuroanatomy class.

But Mrs. Woodson listens intently, her eyes fixed on O'Brien.

"As part of today's evaluation," he says. "I'm going to press on Mrs. Woodson's Main Nerve, and see if she has a seizure. That's why I've asked you two to be here, in case I need your help." He then begins pressing forcefully on the fictitious nerve and, right on cue, Mrs. Woodson begins moaning and wailing, stiffly extending her arms and legs, then jerking and flailing in a gathering crescendo. Finally, she howls and yodels as though she is in the grip of a colossal orgasm.

"That's it!" O'Brien exclaims. "Seizures of the Main Nerve. Rare, but there it is. I'll have to discuss this with my attendings." O'Brien buzzes about the room in irrepressible triumph.

As Andy and I leave Mrs. Woodson's room we do our best to stifle our laughter. "The fictitious Main nerve."

"What a wacko," I say.

"Mrs. Woodson?"

"Both of them."

PHILIP B. DOBRIN, M.D.

CHAPTER 13

HEAD TRAUMA

We finish evening rounds at six-thirty. Andy and Estelle leave the hospital, while our medical student, Eric, and I remain on call for the night. After we make a quick stop in the cafeteria for some vulcanized chicken, we retreat to the nurses' station with our three-by-five cards. We begin ordering blood tests, x-rays, and filling out consent forms to prepare for tomorrow's procedures.

After we've completed our tasks, Eric and I retreat to the call rooms. I phone home to say goodnight to my wife and kids, and get myself ready for a night of neurosurgical calls.

"Don't hesitate to call me," Andy says before he leaves. "Call me with anything, no matter how trivial the question seems, no matter how late the hour."

He and Barney Wilson must have gone to the same school—exhorting the junior residents during the first years of residency. I'll bet they remember how unsure they were during their first nights on call.

I take off my lab coat and shoes, and prop myself up in bed. Tonight I'm going to read about lumbar disc disease before I close my eyes. I make an oath to myself that I will do it, an inviolable promise.

At one a.m., I am awakened by the sounds of activity in the call room next to mine. I hear a woman's sibilant speech and a man's muffled laughter. I have no idea to whom these voices belong, but it really doesn't matter for they soon become silent and are replaced by a rhythmic assessment of the call room's bed springs.

At two a.m., I'm awakened again by a call from the Emergency Room asking me to come see a patient with possible head trauma. I'm still propped up in bed with the Neurosurgery textbook open in front of me, still on the first page of the section on lumbar disc disease. So much for well-intentioned promises. I rouse Eric, and the two of us walk down to the ER together. There we meet Mr. and Mrs. Morris.

Mr. Morris is a sixty year-old accountant, comatose, breathing sonorously.

"We were at home," Mrs. Morris tells us. "He was up on a step ladder in the kitchen when he lost his balance, fell and hit his head on the corner of a kitchen cabinet." She points to his right temple. "I told him not to get up on that ladder at his age, but he's so damn stubborn. He never listens to me. Just last week I was telling him..."

"Did he lose consciousness?" I ask, interrupting her.

"He did. Right away I called 911. By the time the ambulance got there, he was awake again, but he was confused. Not at all like him..."

"how long would you guess he was unconscious?"

"Five, maybe ten minutes. I'm not sure. It seemed a lot longer."

"Just when did all this happen?"

"Three or four hours ago."

Nikki, the night nurse in the ER, tells us that when Mr. Morris arrived at the hospital, the doctor working in the ER ordered skull films.

"I'd like to see them," I say, "Even though they seldom rule in, or rule out, a fracture."

"At first he was awake and alert," Nikki says. "But after about four hours of observation, he lapsed into coma." That's when the ER doctor called you guys."

"All I know about head trauma is what I've read in textbooks," I tell Eric, but this guy looks like the real thing. The first episode of loss of consciousness is probably due to a concussion, and the second is due to bleeding in the skull, putting pressure on the brain.

As a first step, I examine Mr. Morris's neck, even though the doctor working in the ER already examined him. There is no evidence of a neck injury. Moreover, Mr. Morris has been active and has rotated his neck in the ER. Next, Eric and I examine the unconscious Mr. Morris and find a dilated pupil on the right, a so-called blown pupil, and a sign of pressure on the optic nerve. His left eye reacts normally. We test motor reflexes in his arms and legs with our rubber reflex hammers. His reflexes seem weaker on the injured side and stronger than normal on the left side, but I'm not sure; I've never tested reflexes in an unconscious patient before.

I call Andy at home, awakening him from a deep sleep. He sounds groggy and persistently somnolent as I reiterate the history and physical findings.

Suddenly, he is wide awake. "Sounds like an epidural bleed," he says. "I'm on my way, but don't wait for me to get things started. Call the OR, and tell them we need to be on the table in twenty minutes. The same goes for Anesthesia. And of course, you had better call Heineken, and let him know. He's the attending on call for tonight. And if there's going to be any kind of delay in the OR, tell the nurses in the ER to be sure they've got the instruments we need to drill burr holes there. Time is critical."

"And get a chest x-ray so the anesthesiologists will feel confident about his lungs. Otherwise, they will demand a film after I get there, and that will slow everything down."

"I will."

"Put a Foley catheter in his bladder, and start him on mannitol. It will make him urinate and should lower his cerebral pressure. That should give some protection to the brain, at least temporarily. One more thing," he adds. "Is he on an anticoagulant—coumadin or heparin, or even aspirin?"

How dumb of me—I never thought to ask. It's a

good thing to know, whether or not someone has had a cerebral bleed, especially if you're going to be drilling holes in their head. I send Eric back to the family to find out if he's on any so-called blood thinners. He's back in a flash. Shaking his head no.

"He's not on any anticoagulant." I tell Andy.

"Good," he says. "Write up a History and Physical, admit him, get the consent forms signed, and let's roll."

I call the OR and Anesthesia, and they assure me that they'll be ready in twenty to thirty minutes. I also call Dr. Heineken at home to tell him about Mr. Morris. He says that he'll be in, but he sounds so sleepy I'm afraid he may not even remember that I called him.

Mrs. Morris is the patient's wife and next of kin. I describe the likely injury her husband has sustained, and the need to control the bleeding.

She listens half-heartedly, tearful and distracted.

I ask her to sign the consent forms permitting us to do the surgery and administer blood, if it becomes necessary.

"Can't we just watch him for a few hours, and see if he wakes up?"

"Mrs. Morris," I explain with growing exasperation. "I know you would like to wait to see if the fall tore a blood vessel on the surface of your husband's brain. But we must control the bleeding as quickly as we can."

She looks squarely at me. "Who will do the surgery?"

"The Chief of Neurosurgery and the senior resident. I'll be there to help, but they will do the surgery and make all the decisions."

"All right," she says reluctantly. "How soon?"

"Now, as soon as we can."

With the help of the ER staff, we secure Mr. Morris to a gurney. We wheel him to the X-ray department to get a chest film, then onto the elevator to go to the operating suite on the second floor. As we push open the swinging doors to the OR, I realize that I have taken charge, and I'm acting like an honest-to-God neurosurgeon when in fact, I don't have the slightest idea of what to do next. The OR nurses guide me and I follow their lead, but I'm enormously relieved when Andy comes sailing in through the swinging doors to examine Mr. Morris. He checks his pupils, assesses his reflexes and feels for a depressed skull fracture. There's nothing to be felt. I'm relieved because I completely forgot to examine him for a depressed skull fracture.

"Good diagnosis," he says.

I thank him, even though it actually was he who made the diagnosis, not I—and he did it over the telephone. You can't beat the experience of seven years of head trauma to know what you're doing.

"Did you talk to the family?" Andy asks.

"I did. And I got the consent."

"And the chest film?"

"We got it."

"Good, let's scrub."

Andy, Eric and I scrub at the sink outside the operating room while the anesthesiologist and OR crew prepare Mr. Morris for surgery.

"Looks like a classic epidural bleed," Andy says, soapy water running down his forearms. He turns toward Eric. "The first loss of consciousness was from hitting his head. We call it a concussion. It's what happens to football players and boxers when they get hammered. It's from jarring and bruising of the brain. That usually lasts only a few minutes. The awake period that follows the concussion is called the lucid interval as the brain recovers from the acute injury.

"The coma that happens next is different. We think it is from bleeding inside the skull. As blood accumulates, it presses on the brain and the nerves that regulate the eye. That's why we look for a blown pupil."

Eric nods while I take it all in. I've heard all this before, but it's so much more meaningful when I have an actual patient with a problem, rather than to just read about it in a textbook.

"We could take him down to x-ray," Andy says. "And call

in the interventional radiologist to do an angiogram to prove that there's a bleed, but that would take a lot of valuable time. We are making the diagnosis based on clinical signs."

He turns to me. "By the way, what about the skull films?"

"Oh, the skull films. I completely forgot about them. I'm embarrassed to tell you this, but with all the rushing around, I never got to see them. I guess they're still in the ER."

"You guess they're in the ER?" Andy nods his head incredulously. He turns to Erik. "Stop scrubbing," he says. "Go down to the ER and bring up the films."

"There is no point ordering x-rays if you're not going to look at them." Andy says.

I want to tell Andy that I was scrambling, trying to get everything organized and move the patient into the OR as he had directed me to do, that I never ordered the skull films in the first place, that the doctor working in the ER had done so. But I don't say any of those things because he's right; we had the films, and I should have looked at them. Andy's irritation with me seems to pass. Or perhaps it's just concealed.

After scrubbing for five minutes, we enter the operating room, gown and glove, and then drape the patient, and Andy drills two small burr holes above the temple to relieve the pressure that blood is exerting on the brain. Then he quickly makes a semi-circular scalp flap, and removes a disc of skull, the same way he did in Mrs. Hanson and Mrs. Willibrand, the patients who had the brain tumors. As he lifts the disc of skull off the brain, a few cubic centimeters of blood ooze out under pressure. Then we encounter a jellied mass of partially-clotted blood. Andy's over-the-phone diagnosis was indeed correct. He flushes out the opening, then identifies a bleeding artery, and clips it. Now the pressure on the brain is relieved.

I take a moment to stare down at the blood-stained gray convoluted folds of Mr. Morris's exposed brain. It is a mysterious instrument, the brain, the repository of his mind and memory, and all his personal past. Who knows what and how information is stored there. It is a precious past, one that may no longer exist in physical reality, but remains alive and vivid in this man's memory.

My thoughts are interrupted when Dr. Heineken bursts into the room, massive and startling in his glaring white scrubs. Eric is with him, clutching Mr. Morris's skull films to his chest. Dr. Heineken puts the films up on the view box in the operating room, and we squint and shift our positions to here and there to examine them.

"This might be a skull fracture here," Dr. Heineken says, pointing to a fine line on the film. "But it's hard to be sure. If it is, it's a hairline fracture. You'd never be able to feel it. In any case, it's right below where Andy opened the skull—a classic epidural bleed."

Heineken does not scrub, but he remains in the room, watching Andy work. Heineken puts an attending note in the chart, and says that he will join us for morning rounds, after we've finished the case.

As we close, I help by doing whatever Andy asks me to do—hold a retractor to pull back on the scalp, clip the cut edge of the incision where it is trickling a tiny rivulet of red blood, and cut a suture that was used to control a pesky bleeder. None of it requires complex skills—a high school student could do it. But the experience and wisdom knowing when to make the diagnosis, and the decision to operate based on that experience, was Andy's not mine. Nevertheless, right now, I feel less like an interested visitor and more a part of the neurosurgical team.

CHAPTER 14

HEART SURGERY SERVICE

We are in the hall outside the ICU. "It's hard to believe," I tell Lenny, "but my three months as a resident on Neurosurgery are almost over. Cardiothoracic Surgery is next."

"Cardiothoracic Surgery is next for me too," he says.

I feel a momentary wave of anxiety when I think of working side-by-side with the highly-touted always-right never-wrong Lenny Goldstein. He really is a smart guy, causing the rest of us to pall by comparison. He's the kind of surgeon you would want to have operating on you if you had to have surgery. Nothing seems to faze him; everything seems to be simple and fits his often-used description as a *piece of cake.*

Strictly speaking, Cardiothoracic Surgery means surgery of the heart, lungs, chest and esophagus. But with the current developments in cardiac surgery, it mostly means operations on the heart.

***

It's nearly six o'clock in the morning. Lenny and I stand outside the ICU where a whole new cast of characters await us. There are three attending heart surgeons, three residents (including Lenny and myself), and a Cardiothoracic Surgery Fellow. A Fellow is someone who takes an additional year or two of specialized training after completing the five years of residency on General Surgery. That all adds up to a lot of manpower, and I have to wonder if all that is really necessary.

Dr. Abraira is the Chief attending on the Cardiothoracic Surgery service. He's in his early fifties with glossy black hair combed straight back, a calm imperturbable voice, and gold-rimmed glasses. He projects a self-assured bearing. Originally from a Spanish-speaking country, he speaks with a lofty aristocratic flair. He is reputed by some to be the most skilled surgeon in the medical center.

"He really is remarkable," the Cardiothoracic Surgery Fellow standing beside me whispers. "Wait till you see him in the operating room. He never hurries, but always seems to finish before anyone else. Because of the phenomenal amount of money the Cardiovascular Surgery group brings into the university, he also gets just about everything he asks for."

Dr. Abraira's most experienced associate is Dr. Kevin McCarthy, a tall, wide, red-haired Irishman who is said to be impatient, volatile and predictably unpredictable. But he also is reputed to be extremely skilled in the operating room. "Great hands" is what I've heard. Rumor has it that he can precisely run a suture line on the back side of a vessel, even when it is out of direct vision. And he is fast, really fast. But I've also been warned by the other residents to steer clear of him, if I can. A guy like that can get riled up and bite your head off over nothing.

The third member of the attending staff is Dr. Jose Martinez—quiet, compellingly handsome with dark hair and dark eyes, and small, sculptured features. He's overflowing with Latin charm, and I've seen more than one young nurse melt under his gaze. He also is supposed to be a wizard in the operating room, but I guess you have to be if you're going to be a heart surgeon.

In addition, there are three General Surgery

residents rotating on the Cardiovascular Surgery service doing the daily work. The first is my acquaintance, Lenny Goldstein. The second General Surgery resident is Ken Wharton. He is a tall, easy-going guy, but he is in his third year of General Surgery, and is openly resentful about being assigned to the Cardiothoracic Surgery service at such an advanced stage of his training. He complains that none of us will be getting much hands-on operative experience.

"I'll be honest with you," he mutters. "They're using us for slave labor."

Resentful or not, I hope he bears his share of the workload.

Finally, there's the Cardiovascular Surgery Fellow, Walter Crane. He's a blond-haired, long-faced man who wears milk bottle-thick eye glasses that always seem to be staring at you. The best place to find him is in the hospital, dressed in scrubs, in the OR checking on one patient or another, clomping around in loose penny loafers. He is in his seventh year of training. As with most fellowships, he is expected to act as first assistant on as many scheduled cases and emergency procedures as he can, helping the attendings, and accumulating surgical experience. Walter can be found strolling through rounds holding a polystyrene coffee cup with no more than a few thimblefuls of coffee, so little that it doesn't even darken the bottom of the cup.

"Why don't you take a full cup of coffee?" I ask him

"I would," he says. "But I never know when I'm going to be able to sleep, and when I'm going to have an emergency case."

What he says makes sense. "You might say that I want to be awake, but I don't want to face reality." No one laughs. I know he really means it.

Three attendings, three residents, and a cardiacthoracic surgery fellow; that's a lot of manpower. I wonder if all that is really necessary, or is this just a power play by the Cardiovascular Surgery service?

It is precisely six a.m., Drs. Abraira, McCarthy, and

93

Martinez, the three attending surgeons, emerge from the Surgical ICU to greet us outside the intensive care unit area. They earnestly look at each one of us in the eye as they reach out to shake our hands. Dr. Abraira has a pronounced stoop, the legacy, I suspect, of having spent thousands of hours bent over patients in the operating room.

"Today should be easy" he says. We have scheduled no surgery so we can all become acquainted, and go over our routines. Let's begin by visiting the ICU."

The Surgical ICU is a large, noisy room with ten beds, five lining two opposing walls. Each bed is surrounded by a forest of dangling IV lines.

Of the ten beds in this room, eight are occupied by patients recuperating from cardiac surgery. The other two beds are for General Surgery patients or Neurosurgery patients, whoever occupies them first.

Dr. Abraira addresses us about the utilization of beds. "One of your responsibilities is to always keep eight beds occupied by our patients. If a patient is to be transferred out to the floor, stall and keep them here to protect the bed until we have someone else ready to take his place. Otherwise, General Surgery or Neurosurgery will grab the bed, and our patients will have no place to go. That means we will not be able to do their heart surgery, and many of the patients may not survive without it. Remember, after cardiac surgery, our patients don't go to the Recovery Room like other services—they come directly here, to the ICU. So we must be able to receive them."

Clearly, Dr. Abraira views coronary artery surgery as the most important surgical procedure; considering how many people die of coronary artery disease each year, his argument may be right. Or is it simply a reflection of power, who controls the beds and therefore the operating room time?

Dr. McCarthy snorts at the notion that another service might want to use one of Cardiothoracic Surgery's beds. "They've already got two beds," he says.

"What more do they want?" He projects the imperious attitude of the Cardiothoracic Surgery group, but displays none of Dr. Abraira's gracious aristocratic flair.

"Actually," Dr. Abraira says, "I've been talking with the hospital administrator about getting us more beds, an ICU just for Cardiothoracic Surgery. I'd like to see twenty-four beds."

A twenty-four bed ICU devoted entirely to cardiac surgery! Where would they find the skilled nurses to staff it? At three shifts a day plus vacations and sick leave, Cardiothoracic Surgery would need well over a hundred skilled ICU nurses, and who knows how many residents. I had no idea what expansionist maneuvers take place behind the scenes at University Hospital. But so be it; let the various services devour each other, if that's what they want to do; we residents are mere spectators, here to work and learn, not get caught up in all the internecine politics.

The seven of us—the three attendings, three residents and the fellow—stroll through the ICU, reviewing each patient. Then we walk through the step-down unit, examine their wounds, and check their data sheers. This lists their heart rhythms, their vital signs, lab data, intravenous fluid intake, chest tube output and urine output. I write everything on my three-by-five index cards, while Lenny simply commits all the abnormal values to memory. He also notes the appropriate actions to correct them. I have no idea how he can do that, but it seems to be a routine, effortless activity for him.

Each patient sits upright, waiting for a kind word and an assuring pat from their attending surgeon. Family members visiting loved ones jump to their feet when we stop for a moment. Their eyes are locked on Drs. Abraira, McCarthy and Martinez. These are not just heart surgeons; these are *their* heart surgeons who performed magical feats in their now closed chests.

We also meet the ICU nurses who are among the most skilled and knowledgeable caregivers in the hospital. Their hours are long, and their work is demanding, but they seem to love it. They are experts and are almost haughty in their self-confidence. In fact, other nurses around the hospital resent them for their cocky attitude, but it seems to be well-deserved.

The head nurse is Cathy Mayor, a middle-aged, no-nonsense, dishwater blonde who rides herd on her restless crew, and takes care of scheduling and administrative responsibilities to boot. The MAYOR of the ICU someone calls her. She joins us for our walk through the ICU, and from her remarks it's evident that she and her crew thoroughly know each patient's clinical status.

"This is Mr. Green," Cathy gestures to Harold Green. "He's breathing on his own, and his respiratory parameters are good. I think we can start weaning him off the off the ventilator today."

Lenny nods in agreement.

"The next patient," Cathy says, "Is Mr. Horowitz. His potassium is chronically low. We need to correct that promptly."

Walter nods in agreement then takes note of it.

Lenny grabs Mr. Horowitz's chart and, on the spot, writes definitive corrective IV orders.

"No point fooling around with his labs," he says. "We might as well correct them right now."

"The next two patients are Mr. Waldo and Mrs. Mareaux," Cathy says. "They will be ready to give up their chest tubes today."

Walter writes a reminder note to himself to pull the tubes.

Having someone to carefully watch over the patients in the ICU while we are tied up in the operating room is a wonderful advantage. It is as though the cardiothoracic surgery service had a well-informed extra ICU resident. And anyone can see how completely the cardiac surgery attendings trust and rely on the nurses' judgment.

Every now and then, we see a nurse walking with a patient who is dressed in street clothes. Cathy Mayor explains that these patients are scheduled for cardiac surgery in the next week, and that their clinical experience will be less overwhelming if they have been introduced to the ICU before surgery.

***

"Cardiac surgery is complicated," Dr. Abraira says as we stroll through the ICU. "But we do the same operation so often, it's become routine. Last year, the nurses developed standing orders for the patients in the ICU, so after surgery, you don't have to create detailed post-op orders. All you must do is sign the preprinted orders sheet and give it to the nurses. You may have to make a few adjustments here and there—like insulin orders for diabetics, and heparin for patients with a newly implanted valve—but pretty much everything is taken care of for you. But," he reminds us, "you do have to write daily progress notes in each patient's chart so we document their clinical progress. There are no preprinted progress notes."

Several of the patients who had surgery in the last forty-eight hours have one, or a pair, of garden hose-size clear plastic tubes protruding from their chests—so-called chest tubes.

"We insert these in the OR," Dr. Abraira says, "just before we close the chest. We want to capture any oozing in the closed chest, to prevent it from accumulating and restricting filling of the heart. They must always be on suction." He points to four patients with suction devices bubbling noisily at the sides of their beds.

"When the drainage falls to less than 100 cc in 12 hours, we remove the chest tubes. That's usually within 48 hours of surgery. You can come back later with Walter, and he'll show you how to take them out."

I stand dazzled by the active efficiency of the ICU, but I can't get over how much this place feels and sounds like a production line in a busy factory.

After we finish in the ICU, the three attending surgeons leave to examine angiograms in the cardiac cath lab for tomorrow's surgery. But before they go, Dr.

Abraira brings up an all-together too familiar subject.

"I know you've heard all this before, but please keep up with your discharge summaries. When we get busy, you will have so many discharges, it will be impossible to remember one patient from another. Do your dictations every night, before you go home."

Walter has a faint smile. "Did you hear what Dr. Abraira said? Before you go home. That's *if* you go home."

Everyone laughs politely, but I'm not certain that remark was intended to be funny.

We now leave the ICU, and Walter takes us to Three East. This is a unit that is separate from the ICU. It is a ward of single and double-bed rooms which serves as a step-down unit for the ICU. Post-operatively, patients are transferred from the ICU to Three East when they are stable, and soon will be discharged to home. Each bed is equipped with a heart monitor that continuously transmits the electrocardiograms (EKG's) to a console in the nurses' station.

"We have twenty-six beds here," Walter says. "We see every patient every day. The cardiologists come by to see them as well, so be sure to read the notes the cardiologists put in the charts. They often have good ideas about changing the patient's medications. But remember, as long as the patients are here, they're ours; we write the orders, not the cardiologists."

Still, I am overwhelmed by the sheer volume of the work—eight to ten patients in the ICU plus twenty-six patients in the step-down unit. And, of course, two or three of us are conscripted to assist in surgery at any given time, so we are not freely available to look after the post-op patients.

"When the patients are ready," Walter says, "We send them home from here, from the step-down unit. If they have an abnormal heart rhythm or cardiac pumping problem, we sometimes transfer them to Cardiology, but we don't have to do that very often.

"The cardiology residents really don't want our patients because then they get stuck having to dictate the discharge summaries." Walter chuckles. His days of heavy paperwork are behind him—as long as we are around to do it for him.

I take a minute to review my notes on patient flow. Patients are referred by their family physician to a cardiologist because of suspected heart symptoms. The cardiologist does some testing, including a treadmill and, if indicated, a cardiac catheterization to visualize the coronary arteries. If there is critical narrowing of the coronary vessels, the patient is referred to the cardiothoracic surgeons for an operation. The idea is to prevent a heart attack or, if necessary, treat a heart attack.

After surgery, the patients remain in the ICU until they are stable. This usually requires about 72 hours. While they are there, they are our responsibility. When they are stable, we transfer them to the step-down unit, i.e., to Three East. When they are stable on Three East, we discharge them to home. After that, the cardiac surgeons see them once or twice in clinic to check their wounds. Then they are sent back to their cardiologist, who either keeps them for their cardiac problems, or refers them back to their family physicians. It all forms a big loop.

"How many cases do you do a day?" I ask Walter.

"Oh, three, maybe four. Sometimes five when we're really busy or have an emergency. About a thousand cases a year. Abraira almost never refuses the cardiologists."

"Where do you get all the beds for these patients?"

"That's your job," Walter says.

It sounds impossible. You can't just shuffle patients out the door because you need their bed. But I will not be the first resident to work here, so I'll figure something out.

I stand aside for a moment and recount my responsibilities: Assist in the operating room, manage the patients in the ICU, care for the patients on Three East, discharge three or four patients a day, and dictate their discharge summaries.

Now I see why the service requires all this manpower.

It's a busy factory that bypasses clogged arteries. These are required to deliver blood to feed the heart muscle. And for the powerful people who own the factory, it's a life-saving money-making business. It's also clear that the cardiac surgeons want to accommodate the cardiologists to maintain a constant stream of patients. Every one at every level wants to keep his or her customers happy.

Lenny is with us, but he hasn't said a word. He stands off to one side, taking it all in. I wonder what he thinks of all this.

"You can come back to Three East later to see the patients," Walter says. "They'll need progress notes in their charts. Sometimes it gets to be a long day, but you'll learn to cope."

He sits down on the corner of an unoccupied patient bed, takes off his milk bottle-thick glasses and polishes them with the corner of his lab coat. "In a couple of days we'll be getting the medical students—they'll help by writing progress notes and keeping up with the scut work. But don't forget; you guys have to read and countersign their notes."

"By the way," Walter adds. "Dr. Abraira doesn't mind the students coming into the OR to watch the surgery, but he doesn't like them to scrub in the OR or take care of the patients in the ICU. Those patients are acutely ill, and caring for them is your responsibility."

"Hey!" he says. "It's not too late to hit the cafeteria. There might be enough time to grab a quick lunch before they close. You'd best take advantage of it while you can. It may be your only chance for the next three months."

For a moment I think of hungry Nathan. I wonder how he's doing, no doubt, eating lunch somewhere.

***

After lunch, Walter leads us back up to the ICU. "Come along," he says. "And I'll show you how to take out chest tubes."

We follow him down the hall as he instructs us. "The lungs are held open because they stick to the inside of the chest wall by surface tension. The chest tubes must always be on suction—always, always, always. Or else they'll let air into the chest cavity. This will permit the lung to collapse, a pneumothorax.

"On post-op day two or three, whenever the output from the chest tube is less than 100 cc over 12 hours, we remove the tube, and seal the incision with Vaseline-covered gauze. To keep air from entering the chest while we're pulling out the chest tube, we sit the patients up and have them exhale against a closed glottis. Like when they're straining on the toilet. That's what I tell them, and they always understand what I want them to do.

Walter demonstrates how we remove a chest tube from a patient, Mr. McKeen, one of a roomful of ICU patients. "Keep straining," Walter urges. "Keep straining...keep straining..." And, with a continuous motion, he pulls the tube out from between Mr. McKeen's ribs. Even as the tube is moving outward, he applies the Vaseline-smeared gauze to the opening in the skin to seal the opening.

Mr. McKeen yelps involuntarily as Walter pulls the tube.

It's simple enough, as long as the patient keeps straining and doesn't take a breath at the wrong time.

"What do we do next?" Walter asks.

"Get a chest x-ray," Lenny answers.

"Bright boy! To be sure that the lung hasn't collapsed." Walter points to a radiology technician entering the ICU with a clumsy, motorized portable X-ray machine. "That's why the x-ray technician comes up every morning, to take a chest film of each of the ICU patients, and to take a film whenever we take out a chest tube. It's a daily ritual. And how do we verify that we didn't give the patient a substantial pneumothorax while we're waiting for the chest x-ray?"

"Use our stethoscope to listen for breath sounds," I say.

PHILIP B. DOBRIN, M.D.

"Right on," Walter says.

Each of us then takes a turn removing the chest tubes from a patient. Walter hovers over us, directing the sequence of steps. "By the way," he adds, "in case you're wondering, when you pull the tube out, it hurts for just a moment or so, but it's not too bad."

Not too bad. That's what he says because it's being done to someone else, and not to him. In spite of his assurances, I notice that each patient cries out and jumps involuntarily as we pull out the tubes. I make a silent resolution that when I'm doing this; I'm going to order a dose of intravenous Demerol to deaden the pain a few minutes before I pull the tube.

"By the way," Walter asks. "What do you do if you do get a pneumothorax?"

"Put in another chest tube," Lenny answers.

Of course. I have inserted and removed chest tubes in the laboratory, but I never actually inserted a chest tube in a real live patient. After a few minutes, the x-ray technician brings us the portable chest films taken after we pulled the tubes. I put them up on the view box on the wall of the ICU, and we start searching for evidence of a pneumothorax. Walter looks on.

"No point ordering x-rays, if we're not going to look at them." I say. Andy, the senior resident in Neurosurgery, would be proud of me.

"Hey, that's a good line," Walter says. "I've got to remember that. I'll use it on the medical students."

Walter leaves us to go to clinic. Lenny, Ken and I spend the afternoon reviewing the patient charts and meeting all the patients, those in the ICU and those on Three East. It's hard to separate the patients because they all had similar symptoms when they were admitted, and they all had more or less the same operation. Only the specific location of arterial narrowing is different from one patient to another. This place really is a factory—a high stakes enterprise—but a factory, nevertheless.

102

CHAPTER 15

CORONARY ARTERY BY-PASS

Today is our second day on the Cardiac Surgery service, our first operating day. Walter, Lenny, Ken and I are in the ICU seeing the patients who had surgery in the past few days. We examine their incisions, assess their vital signs, and review their lab data. We adjust some of the IV fluid rates, and we write a brief progress note in each patient's chart. I read over my brief note.

Post-op Day Three: Doing well. Wounds clean and dry. No fever. White blood count elevated to 11,500.

Chest tube drainage 75 cc over past 12 hours.

Plan: pull chest tube this morning. If stable, will transfer to 3 East.

Philip Dobrin, M.D.

At seven o'clock, Ken and I leave the ICU to go to the operating room to assist the attendings, while Lenny remains in the ICU to remove the chest tubes from the ICU patients who have low chest tube output. Writing progress notes is one thing on General Surgery or Neurosurgery where there are just a few patients; but it is quite a different task where there are 25 or 30 post-op patients. My three-by-five cards will be doing yeoman's service, and will require frequent updating during the day.

In the late afternoon, Walter returns to lead us on rounds and revisit all our hospitalized patients. He examines each patient's chest and groin incisions; listens to their heart, and reviews their lab data. Using this information, he identifies four patients whom we should be able to discharge tomorrow. I take careful notes as we chug along, the pockets of my lab coat bulging with stacks of three-by-five cards, my pager, my stethoscope, a pocket flashlight and some hard candies.

After evening rounds, we have about an hour's worth of work left to do. Lenny is on call tonight, so Ken Wharton and I help him by getting the consent forms signed for tomorrow's surgery.

I take a consent form to a Mr. Martucci, a cheerful, roly-poly Italian grocer with sparkling eyes and a voluminous white moustache. According to his chart, he started having chest pains about a month ago. At his wife's insistence, he saw his family doctor. From there he was referred to a cardiologist who performed a treadmill test and a cardiac catheterization. The tests show narrowing in each of the three main coronary arteries, as I explain this to Mr. Martucci.

"Too much prosciutto," he says with a wide mustachioed grin.

"Chest pains, and shortness of breath with exertion— are all signs that there are blockages in the coronary arteries, and that a heart attack may not be far off."

Mr. Martucci is interested in what I have to say, but Mrs. Martucci is especially attentive, hovering over us like a concerned parent. She's an unsmiling, gray-haired lady dressed in a plain black shift, with a few strands of silvery gray hair on her shoulders.

"Tomorrow," I say to Mr. Martucci. "We're going to take a segment of vein from your leg, and use it to bypass the blockages in the arteries in your heart. This should make you feel better, and may lessen your chances of having a heart attack."

Mr. Martucci nods.

"If the blockages are in his arteries," Mrs. Martucci asks, "why are you using a vein? Shouldn't you be using an artery?"

"That's a good question. We use veins because they deliver adequate blood flow and they tend to stay open. There are plenty of veins available. In fact, we have veins to spare, but we don't have arteries to spare."

Mrs. Martucci stares at me; she doesn't seem convinced.

I return to her husband. "We need for you to read and sign this consent form. It gives us permission to do the operation."

Mrs. Martucci gazes at me suspiciously. "You brought the consent form for us to read and sign, but isn't Dr. Abraira going to be doing the surgery? That's why we came here."

"Oh yes, of course," I say. "Cardiac surgery is complicated business, and it works best with a team effort. We're going to help Dr. Abraira."

I'm quoting the chief, and the more I hear the words, the more convincing they sound. Even to me. Besides, they speak the truth.

At last, Mrs. Martucci appears to be satisfied.

Her husband slips on his glasses, and takes the consent form. It's a medico-legal document originally written in simple English by the ICU nurses, and later obfuscated by the hospital lawyers.

Mr. Martucci starts to read it, his lips moving silently as he struggles with the text and its unfamiliar medical terms.

"Oh, just sign it, Rocco," Mrs. Martucci says impatiently. "You don't know what you're reading anyway."

He signs the form and hands it back to me.

"Do you have any questions?" I ask Mr. Martucci.

Before he can answer, Mrs. Martucci shakes her head 'no,' and dismisses me with a wave of her hand.

***

Dr. Abraira, Walter and I stand at the sink outside the Operating Room, scrubbing our hands and forearms, watching the activities in the operating room through the large observation window above the sink.

Everyone is quiet as we watch the anesthesiologists work on Mr. Martucci. He lies on the operating table under a bundle of IV lines that are inserted into veins in his arms and neck.

He is anesthetized, and the anesthesiologist is securing a tube in his airway by taping it to his face and neck. Sitting beside the operating table is a file cabinet-size bypass pump on large wheels. A pump technician is camped on a stool beside it reading Road and Track magazine. He looks bored, waiting for the case to begin. He does this every day, all day long, reading about the latest Ferrari until his skills are required.

After five minutes, Dr. Abraira stops scrubbing and drops his brush in the sink. We all do the same and follow him into the operating room, like chicks following a mother hen. No one says a word. After we have gowned and gloved, Dr. Abraira and Walter drape the patient.

After making a superficial skin incision down the middle of Mr. Martucci's chest with a scalpel, Dr. Abraira uses a pneumatic saw that looks like a Sears saber saw to split open the chest cavity. He inserts the saw near the bottom of the rib cage in the midline and with a high-pitched whine, saws open the sternum from below his ribs, up through the middle of his chest to just below his neck. It's startling to see a man split open like a walnut for the length of his chest.

Dr. Abraira then inserts a gleaming steel retractor into the opening and extends its arms apart by twisting a crank. As the arms of the retractor slowly are spread the lungs appear, rhythmically filling and retracting with each breath. As the retractor is spread further, Mr. Martucci's heart emerges in the center of his chest between his lungs. His heart is cloaked by its tough surrounding pericardium.

When Dr Abraira opens the pericardium still further, the heart jumps forward like a red, muscular football. It is the color and texture of raw steak, streaked with ribbons of fat that run the length of its surface overlying the course of each coronary artery. Dr. Abraira takes my gloved hand, inviting me to touch the exposed heart. I do so, and I am surprised by how hard it is, as firm as a clenched fist gripping an incompressible sphere of blood. It contracts with mindless regularity, driven by an internal physiological clock. As the heart fills with blood, it elongates until it looks progressively more like a football. Then, with the blink of an eye, it contracts, shortening into a more spherical shape, expelling the blood into the aorta and the pulmonary arteries. Elongating-shortening, elongating-shortening, seventy times a minute, a hundred thousand times a day, thirty million times a year for seventy years. How the sight of this amazing organ must have mesmerized primitive man; it dazzles me, and I was trained in medical school to understand it. Truly, an amazing machine.

Dr. Abraira inserts a catheter, i.e., a slender plastic tube, into Mr. Martucci's atrium, one of the two small cardiac chambers, to capture blood returning to the heart. He places a tie around the atrial tissue, then snugs it around the catheter to be sure it doesn't leak.

He then inserts another catheter into Mr. Martucci's aorta, the large artery through which blood flows out of his heart. These are connected through the bulky bypass pump, a device which both oxygenates and pumps his blood, replacing the function of both his lungs and heart.

Walter shows me how to assemble all the sterile connectors, permitting redirection of blood flow through the bypass pump. The room is now filled with the steady hum of the bypass pump; a droning, comforting sound as technology takes precedence over biology for the next sixty to ninety minutes.

Mr. Martucci's heart continues to beat, but, with all its motion, Dr. Abraira cannot perform the delicate surgery required on the small coronary arteries. To abolish this motion, he applies an electrical stimulus to the surface of the heart. Instantly, the contracting heart loses its regular rhythm, and fibrillates, wriggling like a bag of worms, as thousands of cardiac cells contract without synchronization.

If fibrillation had occurred while Mr. Martucci was standing in his grocery store, his heart would cease to pump blood, and his brain, heart muscle and other organs would be in jeopardy. In fact, his heart and brain would have just minutes to live. But here, with the bypass pump replacing the functions of his lungs and heart, his vital organs are protected, and the delicately trembling heart seems to await the surgeon's hands.

Dr. Abraira quickly identifies the narrowed areas of each coronary artery which he observed yesterday on the cardiac cath lab films. Now, in the operating room, he confirms the location of narrowing by running his fingers over the surface of the coronary arteries." Right here," he says, his gloved fingers resting lightly on one of the coronary vessels. "Do you feel it? Some of the areas of blockage have accumulated calcium, and are stony hard to the touch."

He guides my gloved hand, sliding my fingers along the artery until I feel the hardened area; the location of a calcified, cholesterol-ladened plaque. "Yes—I can feel it!"

If these areas of narrowing were to obstruct blood flow, they would cause an MI, a myocardial infarction, a heart attack—all names for the same life-threatening condition. But now that the location of narrowing has been identified, Dr. Abraira dissects the fat overlying the coronary artery. He does this until the narrowed area of the coronary artery is exposed.

Meanwhile Walter makes an incision in Mr. Martucci's thigh. I assist him as he dissects free a few centimeters of saphenous vein. Segments of this vein will be used as a conduit to bypass the diseased arteries. We tie or clip branches, and lift the dissected vein out of the leg. Walter wraps it in a blanket of saline-soaked gauze and sets it aside in a ordinary, but sterile, plastic kitchen dish. The scrub nurse hands me a curved needle and suture mounted in a needle-holder, and Walter directs me to close the skin incision that he made to obtain the vein. I return to the skills I learned in General Surgery. I can hear Dr. Peterson's voice encouraging me, warning me, admonishing me...

108

"In the next case you will harvest the vein, and I will assist you." Walter says.

Now, Walter gives me an invaluable bit of information. "Don't think of the vein dissection as a trivial part of the operation," he says. "You're cutting across small veins and lymphatic channels that play a role in recapturing fluid from the tissues. Post-op, it's the biggest complaint that patients have—swelling and wound-healing problems in the leg where the vein was removed and the lymphatics were transected. If you know someone who has had bypass surgery, just ask them about what has given them the most discomfort and problems. You have to be very precise the way you close these wounds."

Dr. Abraira and Walter now begin the coronary artery-bypass part of the operation. He takes a segment of the vein that Walter and I harvested and sews one end of the vein to the punched-out area of the aorta. Next, he makes a small opening in the coronary artery, just below the obstructed area, and sews the other end of the vein to the coronary artery. In this way, the excised segment of vein acts as a bridge bypassing the blocked or narrowed areas of the coronary artery. Dr. Abraira uses blue non-absorbable suture (fishing line), so fine and delicate that it seems to disappear as the light on it shifts from moment to moment.

Drs. Abraira and Walter perform this procedure three times, once for each of the three coronary arteries. This is what both laymen and physicians refer to as a "triple bypass."

As they sew these fine vessels, I assist by reaching forward with a small plastic suction tube to capture and control blood spurting from the open coronary arteries as Dr. Abraira sews the vein segment to them. Capturing spilled blood seems like such a trivial part of the operation, but the delicate bypass procedure cannot be done without a clear and unobstructed view. I am pleased to help in any way that I can.

"Help me, boys. Help me," Dr. Abraira says theatrically whenever blood obscures his view. "I cannot do it alone." His accent becomes more pronounced now when he's under pressure. He is good-natured about it, but there is tension in his voice. The longer the patient is on the bypass pump, the greater the post-operative complications he may experience—memory loss, clotting problems among them—as the blood cells are injured by the rollers of the bypass pump.

When the last narrowed artery has been bypassed, Dr. Abraira defibrillates Mr. Martucci's heart with paddles applied directly to the surface of his heart. This is one of the most startling aspects of the operation. It resembles cardiopulmonary resuscitation (CPR), but with the defibrillation paddles discharging an electric shock not through the skin, but directly into his exposed heart. It is as though we are bringing a dead man back to life. When the paddles are discharged, Mr. Martucci's back muscles contract, momentarily lifting him off the operating table. Then he settles back, his heart resuming normal-looking contractions.

As his heart recovers its contractile strength, the pump technician progressively reduces the amount of flow provided by the bypass pump, and increases the portion of flow provided by Mr. Martucci's heart. In just a few minutes, Mr. Martucci's heart will beat independently, free of the pump.

"He has a strong ventricle," Walter says. "Wait till you see some of these patients. Their ventricles are so poor it's a real struggle to wean them off bypass and get them pumping on their own."

Now it is time to finish the operation.

Before closing the chest, Walter inserts two chest tubes, one on each side of the heart. He connects them to a suction device that sits on the floor beside the operating table.

The tubes are placed in the chest to prevent the bloody ooze from accumulating. Then we close the chest. Walter and Dr. Abraira close the midline incision with stout, double-stranded, stainless steel wire sutures that lash together the bony sternum before they are tied. This locks together the two sides of the divided sternum. This is important because an unstable post-operative sternum is difficult to treat and may require re-operation. Lastly, we close the skin. Dr. Abraira encourages me to proceed. "Be careful," he warns. "If the patient doesn't like the looks of his chest wound after surgery, you know who is going to get the blame."

It is a joke, but it's also the truth. After I close the skin, we slide Mr. Martucci off the operating room table and onto a hospital bed. As we roll him into the ICU, the nurses descend upon us, sorting out Mr. Martucci's IV lines, and airway. They immediately begin recording his vital signs, searching for excessive bleeding or excessive chest tube drainage. It is a frenzy of activity as they aggressively fulfill their responsibilities. The nurses have met each of the patients before surgery, and their concern has the flavor of a first name family relationship.

Dr. Abraira stands by, observing the immediate post-operative care, watching for clues of problems such as excessive bleeding from the chest tubes, or a fall in blood pressure. After 15 or 20 minutes, Dr. Abraira leaves to speak with Mrs. Martucci. I can see them as they stand at the doorway to the ICU. I must say that I never expected to see Mrs. Martucci smile, but there it is—something to cheer about.

Eleven o'clock. Four hours have soared by in the operating room, feeling more like twenty minutes. Where has the morning gone?

***

In the ICU, I learn that Lenny is scrubbed on a case with Dr. McCarthy and Ken is scrubbed on a case with Dr. Martinez. This service really is a factory. An ICU nurse tells me that Lenny took care of all the chest tubes and progress notes in the ICU, but he did not get to see the patients on Three East. That dictates what I must do next.

I head to Three East to examine the patients and write discharge orders, prescriptions, and orders for return to clinic. Finally, I must remember to dictate a

111

discharge summary for each of the four or five patients we are going to discharge, but there's no time for that now.

On Three East, I write progress notes and orders for twenty-five patients. I try for efficiency, so I stack all twenty-five charts on a wheeled utility cart, and begin pushing it along, making entries as I visit each patient. I'm reminded of the faded sepia-colored photographs I've seen of my immigrant family on the streets of New York at the turn of the century. They were immigrants from Austria and Russia, bent over their pushcarts, hawking their wares. I am pushing a cart filled with medical charts, and I can only imagine how proud they would be of me.

***

After I've seen just six of our patients, I am interrupted by a page from Walter saying, "Come to the operating room STAT." I abandon the cart to the nurses on Three East and rush to the OR.

Walter is at the scrub sink when I arrive. "The cath lab has an emergency," he says. "They were catheterizing some guy named Anson when he had an MI on the cath table, right in front of them. Abraira is going to do him as an emergency in Operating Room Three."

I change into clean scrubs, spend a vigorous five minutes at the scrub sink, and catch up with Dr. Abraira and Walter at the operating table. They've already opened Mr. Anson's chest when I arrive, and Walter is excising the saphenous vein from the leg in preparation for bypass. Time is critical. If Dr. Abraira can bypass Mr. Anson's occluded coronary arteries soon enough, they may be able to limit the size of the injury done to the heart muscle. Dr. Abraira inserts catheters into the atrium and aorta, connects them to the pump tubing, and fibrillates the heart, just as we had done on Mr. Martucci. But there is no idle chatter, and I am struck by how smoothly and quickly the steps are carried out. With each step in the procedure, the scrub nurse silently anticipates the surgeon's needs for hemostats, needles and needle holders. She offers them even before Abraira reaches for them. He almost never speaks, or even turns his head toward the scrub nurse. He just reaches out. She gives him the instrument he requires.

I notice an area at the apex of the heart, near the end of the "football," that is dusky blue. It is unlike Mr. Martucci's vigorous heart. This patient's heart seems to contract flaccidly, without much strength. The coronary arteries supplying blood to the heart muscle are crucial for the strength of cardiac contraction.

Walter points to a dusky area. "There's the infarct, right there."

I stare, witnessing a heart attack as it is happening. It is a phenomenon that even cardiologists observing changes in the EKG can never see.

Dr. Abraira looks up for a moment, and glares reproachfully at us, apparently distracted by our chatter. Then he returns to his task. He and Walter dissect the fat off the occluded coronary artery, and sew one end of the vein segment to the aorta, the other end of the vein to the coronary artery below the area of occlusion. He is "bypassing" the blocked area of coronary artery, redirecting blood flow around the occluded area. I assist with the suction catheter to keep blood from obscuring the operative field. Moving with unhurried rapidity, Dr. Abraira completes the sewn connections. It is a replication of what we did for Mr. Martucci, but in Mr. Anson's case, there is dramatic urgency.

When Dr. Abraira permits blood to flow to the blood-deprived area, the color of Mr. Anson's heart changes from dusky blue to pink, and then to a luxuriant red.

The lower half of Abraira's face is covered by his surgical mask, but I can see a smile in his eyes.

"You see?" He points to the area. "When tissue has been deprived of blood for a time, it tries to compensate when flow is restored with increased blood flow, even more than normal—hyperemia.

I think of my son after he's been out playing in the cold, and how his ears turn bright red when he comes into the warm house—hyperemia.

We return to the task at hand. Dr. Abraira and Walter now bypass two other areas of coronary narrowing. Then they defibrillate the heart with paddles. At first the heart beats erratically, but gradually it acquires a steady rhythm. The improvement in the vigor of cardiac contractions after bypass is striking. We have re-vascularized the heart, bypassing the narrowed areas of the coronary artery in time.

Dr. Abraira steps back from the table, and unties his gown. His cap and gown are both soaked through with dark perspiration. "Why don't you two close," he says to Walter and me. "I'll put a note in the chart and speak to the family." He takes the chart and sits down on a stainless steel stool, his stoop more pronounced than ever. He could walk out to the doctors' lounge, and give some respite to his tortured back, but he remains near his patient, as if held by an invisible hand.

Meanwhile, Walter and I complete the operation. We insert two chest tubes and close the chest. When Mr. Anson is stable, we slide him off the operating table and onto a hospital bed. Then we wheel him out to the ICU. He is a lucky man, and I have witnessed a near miracle; we actually reversed a heart attack as it was happening. It was as though we were able to make time run backwards. Whether there will be residual damage to his heart remains to be seen, but it appears that much of the area of heart that was in jeopardy has been spared. What a fortunate moment in which to have a myocardial infarction—in a hospital with an available operating room and an unoccupied cardiac surgery team standing by. How many of us will be as lucky as that? By the time we get Mr. Anson into the ICU it is well after five o'clock. Walter, Lenny, Ken and I sit down together for the first time all day. We take a deep breath and review the status of all the patients in the ICU and on Three East. Lenny discharged four of them.

"They were really peeved at having to wait all day to leave here," he says. "I don't think they believed me when I told them we were really busy. I guess they think we spend the day like the young residents on television—drinking coffee and making eyes at the nurses." The four of us share a little laugh.

"Truthfully, I don't blame them for being impatient," Ken says. "But I wonder if they would be so put off if Mr. Anson was one of their relatives."

When we finish the patients on ICU and 3 East, we head to the catheterization laboratory in the basement to get ready for tomorrow. We look at the films taken by the cardiologists during today's cardiac caths anticipating tomorrow's surgeries. All three of our surgical attendings are there, studying the films, locating the areas of blockage, pointing them out for each other and for the rest of us. In one frenetic day, we have become members of the team.

Then we return to the floor to get the consents signed for tomorrow's surgery. There are four scheduled cases—Mr. Ponsiglione, Mr. Rubenstein, Mrs. Palumbo, Mr. Knapp—four faceless patients whom I've never met but whose films I've examined. They all have similar symptoms of angina—heaviness or pain in the left chest with discomfort that radiates down the left arm or up into the left side of the neck with exertion, especially after eating a heavy meal—all signs of insufficiency of coronary blood flow. And they all claim that their symptoms are getting worse. They all were transferred to our service today from Cardiology, and they all are scheduled for coronary bypass surgery tomorrow. All four of them will undergo more or less the same operation, coronary bypass—performed with some slight variations depending on the location of the coronary lesions. From my perspective, they resemble four Mr. Martucci's. The assembly line is rolling.

I'm on call tonight, I have to dictate the discharge summaries for the four patients we sent home from Three East. But first I pay a visit to the cafeteria.

Unfortunately they closed at seven, and the double glass doors are locked as securely as if it were Fort Knox; the cafeteria's liver and onions are safe for now. I trudge down to the vending machines, and make a few gourmet choices that will raise my serum cholesterol to levels higher than those of the patients we're operating on tomorrow.

When I get back to the ICU, I wander into the nurses break room where two nurses sit at a large round table cluttered with old dog-eared copies of Cosmopolitan and People magazine. In the middle of the table there's a flat open box with a few remaining squares of cold pepperoni pizza.

"Help yourself," one of the nurses says. "It's from this afternoon. You can heat it up in the microwave."

It's tempting, but each square of pizza is covered with a thin layer of translucent white cheese that looks remarkably like the atherosclerotic plaques that we've been seeing inside the blocked coronary arteries.

"No thanks," I say. "I'm really not hungry."

CHAPTER 16

CARDIAC ARREST

It is five forty-five in the morning, and I am standing with Ken and Lenny outside the ICU. They are rubbing their eyes and yawning, urging their brains to awaken after a night of undisturbed rest. I'm envious; I'm still awake from yesterday.

"How was it last night," Ken asks.

"Busy," I tell him as I drain the ICU coffee pot. "We had a fifty-five year old guy come in through in the Emergency Room with accelerating angina. The cardiologists took him to the cath lab where they identified areas of insufficient coronary artery blood flow. When the cardiologists were finished, they called us, and we ended up operating all night."

There's a surgical truism that states: the trouble with being on call every other night is that you miss half the good cases. It's a zippy one liner, but it's not so clever when you look out the window and see the dawn of another day coming up to greet you, and you haven't been to bed yet for yesterday.

Last night was my first opportunity to operate with Dr. McCarthy. He's a technically gifted surgeon and absolutely fearless. I watched him dissect and sew a bleeding vein high in the chest where you could barely see the vessel, let alone reach it. He's remarkably skilled, but he can be overbearing.

I kept thinking; when this case is over, McCarthy will go home and go to bed, Mr. Barton, the patient will go to the ICU where he'll be watched by the ICU nurses, and I will have to stand in a corner somewhere to prop myself up and face another day. I guess a lot depends on what we encounter today, and who of us will be able to get some sleep

Walter, the cardiovascular surgery fellow, scrubbed with us last night in his usual role of first assistant. As always, I was second assistant, a helper down near the foot of the operating table.

At about four a.m., Walter looked at me with the most unsettling stare; it actually gave me the shivers. He blinked a few times, then backed away from the operating table until he encountered the tiled wall behind him. Then, with his eyes still wide open and his arms folded across his chest, he slid slowly to the floor.

Dr. McCarthy turned to the circulating nurse. "Check him," he said. "Make sure he's breathing."

I couldn't tell if McCarthy was joking or he really meant it.

The nurse checked Walter's pulse and breathing. "He's alive," she said. "He's just fallen asleep. Then she stood up, put her hands on her hips, and glared at McCarthy with a look that only an irate woman could express, that any dummy with half a brain in his head knows that people fall asleep at four o'clock in the morning. I think the whole thing was lost on McCarthy, but I don't blame him; it was four o'clock in the morning for him, too.

McCarthy looked impatiently at me. His frequently performed operation was becoming a shambles what with the cardiovascular surgery fellow asleep on the floor and a first year resident (myself), acting as first assistant. "Move up," he snapped. "You're first assistant now."

"Me? I can't be first assistant. I've never been a first assistant in all my life."

"Well, look around professor," McCarthy said. "There's nobody here except you and me and a couple of nurses. You have to be first assistant."

McCarthy made a small opening in the atrium with a curved instrument, and he slid a catheter into the opening. Then he passed a fine suture around the catheter with a cuff of atrium to prevent blood from leaking out.

"All right," McCarthy said. "Tie it."

I took up the slack in the suture and pulled firmly to tighten it, but McCarthy wasn't satisfied.

"Tighter," he said.

I tightened the loop.

McCarthy grimaced. "Tighter, or it will leak."

"But I'll break it."

"Tighter."

I pulled the suture tighter.

The room was silent. I cautiously applied increasing tension to the suture until we all heard the inevitable snick as the delicate filament broke. I was sure that snick could be heard in every operating room in the western hemisphere.

"You're untrainable," McCarthy said with disgust. He replaced the suture and tied it himself. He didn't break it.

I stood nonplussed, certain that everyone in the room was secretly laughing at me.

Then McCarthy wrapped a new suture around the atrial cuff.

"Tie it," he said.

I did.

"Tighter."

I pulled up on the suture, which now seemed more fragile than ever.

Look, I wanted to say. The only thing this suture does is squeeze the atrium a little to prevent pesky bleeding while we are doing the bypass. We could use any size suture; in fact, a larger, stronger suture would be even better. And whatever we used, it's going to be discarded at the end of the case, so why don't we use a stronger suture? But I wouldn't dare voice such a common sense suggestion. McCarthy is the experienced heart surgeon, not me. And he didn't ask for my opinion.

"Tighter," McCarthy said.

The muscles in my arms trembled as I struggled to take up the slack in the suture, but not break it. This is no life-death crisis. I just wanted to achieve a simple accomplishment—snugging a loop and tying a knot without breaking the damned suture. Thankfully, it remained intact.

The case went well after that, especially after 10 or 15 minutes passed when Walter came back to life, after having slept on the floor. He scrubbed again and returned to serve as first assistant with whispered apologies for having been away. I was pleased to return to the role of second assistant, and McCarthy seemed to calm down after that.

After we finished the case, McCarthy and I stood in the ICU watching the nurses scramble over his patient, and at that moment he really did feel like my patient. When he could stand it no longer, McCarthy fussed and fiddled with the IVs and chest tubes until the nurses pushed him away, insisting that he was doing their job. He stood beside me, but he kept his eyes on his patient.

"I know you haven't first assisted before," he said. "But you did fine. Everything is challenging the first couple of times you do it and tying those fine sutures can be difficult. They certainly were for me. Why don't you ask the scrub nurse to give you some of those sutures so you can practice tying them around the door knobs in the call room? That's where I learned to tie."

It was nice of him to say all that, but I didn't feel one trace better; not in my wildest dreams could I imagine McCarthy ever struggling with a suture the way I did. But if ever he does, I hope I'll be there to see it. So blustery and assertive that I think he sometimes must burn his bridges in front of him.

***

I can see daylight peeking in through the window of the ICU, and soon it will be time for rounds. We start with the patients in the ICU, but it's hard to concentrate; my eyes simply will not focus. Ken doesn't look much better than he did yesterday. He still has a crushing cold. We're all getting worn ragged by this pace, but I must admit I feel privileged to be part of it. As I learn the steps we take in the operating room, I'm beginning to feel like an active member of the heart surgery team.

"So it wasn't so bad, scrubbing with McCarthy?" Walter says.

"How would you know? You slept through the best part of the case.

"I did? Really? For how long was I out?"

"About a half an hour, but you didn't miss much, certainly nothing worth talking about."

Walter stares at me with a puzzled look

***

At seven o'clock, Walter, Ken and Lenny leave for the operating room, while I remain out of the OR to take care of the ICU patients. I must also look after those patients who are on Three East.

I prepare to pull the chest tubes out of two of the patients in the ICU. But first, I order small intravenous doses of Demerol for pain. That seems to abrogate the discomfort patients feel when we pull out their chest tubes.

When all that has been taken care of, I gather up our newly-arrived medical students and we march over to see the 25 patients we have on Three-East. We load up the wheeled utility cart and start rounds when I get paged. "Dr., please call Edna at extension 2150."

Edna? I don't know anyone named Edna. I call the extension number.

"This is Edna Harmon," the voice on the phone says. "Medical Records. According to our records, you've got almost twenty discharge summaries to do."

I make no effort to conceal my irritation. "Look, I'll do them as soon I can. We're getting killed up here."

"You'd better do them," she warns. "Or the hospital will hold your paycheck."

She sounds like she's scolding a child for having spilled his milk. I'm sure she has no idea what our lives are like.

121

"Hold my paycheck! That would be great. I get to work a hundred ten hours a week in the hospital for free. What a deal. Besides, I read an article somewhere where they said that a hospital can't hold our paychecks and, at the same time, require that we work. Not legally, anyway."

"I don't know about it being illegal," she says. I'm just warning you."

"Well, thanks for the heads up. By the way, I'll bet I'm not the only one on your Bad Boy List. How about Ken Wharton and Lenny Goldstein?"

"Well," she says—I can hear her shuffling papers—"Dr. Wharton has as many incomplete records as you do. I'm going to page him next. But Dr. Goldstein is up to date. He doesn't have a single undictated chart. He manages to stay up. Why can't you guys do it?"

Damn that Lenny. Not one undictated chart!

***

The medical students and I push through rounds on Three East. They are new to the service, so today is especially slow. I write all the orders, read and countersign every note and comment they put in the chart. About the time we finish, Dr. Abraira and Walter complete their case and bring their patient into the ICU. Its remarkable how deceptively quick Abraira is, yet he never seems to rush. I stand for a few moments in the ICU. Dr. Abraira seems unoccupied, so I take the opportunity to ask him about his unhurried efficiency.

He smiles softly. "Basically, it's the same procedures we do, over and over."

"In a way, I guess it is."

"Well, I've given a lot of thought to each step. Sometimes I lie in bed at night, and think about how I can position my hands this way or that to save a little motion. If I can save a second here and a second there, it all adds up."

What he says is true. But, of course, he also has a vast experience. Whether you're a surgeon or a violinist—repetition helps.

***

While we stand talking in the ICU, Walter runs up to say that there's been a cardiac arrest in the cath lab. They have a sixty year old patient who has had a heart attack. They are asking for help from cardiac surgery. Remarkably, my exhaustion vanishes as Walter and I storm down the stairs, cast aside the chairs cluttering our path in the family waiting area, and burst into the cath lab.

There, we find the patient in full cardiopulmonary arrest with no detectable pulse and no spontaneous respirations. An anesthesiologist on the Code Blue Team has placed a tube in the patient's airway, and is ventilating him with a hand-held football-like Ambu-Bag. A cardiology resident bends over the patient, giving closed chest massage, but the patient's EKG reflects persistent ventricular fibrillation. Another cardiology resident administers IV medications.

After a few moments, Dr. Abraira arrives. He stands silently, outlined by the light behind him, as though he were bringing salvation. He stands viewing the chaos. He listens to comments voiced by several of the attendings and residents, but he says he doubts that Cardiovascular Surgery has anything to offer this patient.

Nevertheless, a female cardiologist persists. "If he has any chance at all," she pleads. "It must be now." This cardiologist bears personal responsibility for the patient's outcome and clearly, she is hoping for a miracle. "All right," Dr. Abraira says with a sigh. "Let's see what we can do."

Upon hearing those words, the cardiology residents roll a gurney into the cath lab and transfer the patient onto the wheeled stretcher. He is a heavy man, about two hundred-fifty pounds. *Dead weight.* Then Dr. Abraira directs me to climb onto the gurney, and straddle the patient as though he were a horse. I take over the closed chest massage.

"One and two, and three and four..."

The anesthesiologist accompanying us squeezes the respirator bag intermittently to ventilate the patient. Oxygen hisses from a portable green tank tucked on a rack underneath the gurney. I concentrate on the patient, rhythmically pressing down against his chest and heart to produce at least some blood flow out of his heart to keep his brain and heart muscle alive. Then I release the pressure so his heart can fill with venous blood returning to the heart. Then I press again...

"One and two and three and four..."

A portable EKG monitor is with us on the gurney, next to the patient's head. An iridescent green line sweeps across the screen, but there are none of the deflections generated by a living heart.

Someone pushes the gurney with the patient and me on it, rolling us out of the cath lab, down the hall to the elevator.

"One and two..." Past family members in the waiting area. "How's he doing, doc?" a voice asks.

I don't look up or say a word. This man is dead. "One and two...Look out! We need that elevator. Three and four..." We collide with the closed elevator door; it opens for us. "One and two and three and four..." The doors close. We rise to the second floor, bounce slightly as the elevator door opens, roll out into the hall and race to the operating room." One and two and three and four..."

Into the OR suite, through the swinging doors and into operating room three.

A gowned scrub nurse awaits us beside a tray of instruments. Dr. Abraira appears in cap, mask and gown—scrubbed and ready.

"One and two and three and four ..." We slide the patient onto the operating table, and the anesthesiologists insert intravenous lines in his arms and neck. I move with the patient onto the operating table, and continue the cardiac massage. "Three and four..." When everything is ready, Dr. Abraira directs me to stop the closed chest massage.

I'm breathless and exhausted. I look up at the EKG. It is still hopelessly flat, just the regular blips from the unsuccessful pacemaker.

One of the anesthesiologists takes a syringe with a needle as long as my hand, and injects adrenaline directly into the patient's heart—normally, a jolting stimulus.

No response.

The anesthesiologists inject a second medication directly into the heart, but still there is no response.

Finally, Dr. Abraira shakes his head no. "That's enough," he says. "That's all we can do. We're not going to increase our mortality statistics by operating on a man who is already dead." He turns on his heel and walks briskly out of the room, and everyone but the scrub nurse and I follow close behind.

I start toward the door.

"Oh, no," the scrub nurse says to me. "You can't leave until you take out all those IV lines the anesthesiologists put in. You must sew up the veins. If you don't, he'll leak blood all over the floor, and Housekeeping will kill us."

Housekeeping will kill us!? So it has come to that. I have to please the people that wash the floors.

So here I am, alone in that dismal operating room with a scrub nurse I don't know and a dead patient whom I've never seen before. I take a moment to look at his pallid face—no, I don't know him; he is a complete stranger.

I pull up a stainless steel stool, and spin the seat to raise it to my level. Then the nurse hands me a black, silk suture on a needle-holder and, one by one, I pull out each IV catheter from the patient's arms and neck and sew the vein closed, stanching the flow of dark lifeless blood. I'm operating on a dead man.

Thank God I'm not the cardiologist who has to face that man's family.

***

We make evening rounds early, and we're going to get out by six o'clock. I'm weary, but I'm not the only one. Ken's cold is getting worse. He's lost his voice and his nose is bright red; he looks as bad as I feel. But he's on call tonight, and before we leave, he asks Lenny and

125

me if either of us would be willing to trade call for the night. Ken's a good guy and I'd like to help him out but I haven't slept in two days. And Lenny simply refuses to trade call days.

As I drive home, I think about how unrelenting this life is— exhilarating, but without reprieve, a foot soldier in an endless battle. I don't know how Ken is going to make it through the night so I devise a plan. I will set the alarm at home for early in the morning. After I've had some sleep, I'll call into the hospital to see if Ken needs help.

When I get home, I have dinner, visit briefly with my wife and children, and listen half-heartedly to the reliability problems they are having with the afternoon babysitter. The surgical residency is five long years with twelve-hour days, and in-hospital call every third night. I wonder if my wife and kids will even recognize me by the time this is over. When the kids go to bed, I take a relaxing ten minute shower and collapse into bed while my wife watches television. It's about eight o'clock. Not much of a life, but I wouldn't trade it for the world.

When the alarm goes off at two a.m., I feel as ambitious as a fallen tree trunk. My mind refuses to awaken, and the inside of my mouth tastes like sand. But I've had six uninterrupted hours of sleep. I call the operating room to speak to LeRay, the Operating Room night clerk. I ask her if there is any cardiac surgery going on.

"As a matter of fact, there is," she says. "Neurosurgery's doing a subdural, and Dr. Martinez just started an emergency heart."

I dress and drive to the hospital, struggling to stay awake. I breeze through the ICU and Three East. No problems with bleeding or blood pressure or urine output, or anything else that requires immediate attention.

I change into scrubs, wash my hands at the scrub sink and walk into the operating room where Dr. Martinez, Walter and Ken are in the middle of an emergency coronary bypass.

Ken looks like a ghost. His eyes are red, and his face is as pale as a pan of skim milk.

"You're out of here," I say to Ken, jerking my thumb toward the door. "Everything's quiet in the ICU, and Three East is fine. Just find a bed and start sleeping."

"Bless you," he says. And he's not joking. I know; I've been there myself.

"How about me?" Walter asks enviously.

"And what about me?" Dr. Martinez asks.

"Sorry, guys," I say. "The rest of you have to operate and save lives."

A moment of laughter ripples through the room. Fortunately, the case goes smoothly and we finish in time to catch an hour of sleep before starting morning rounds.

"I'm in no mood to hunt for an open call room," Walter says. "I'll take my hour sitting up in a chair." He takes a seat in the ICU nurses break room. Seconds later, he's snoring like a truck in low gear.

It takes me a few minutes to find an empty call room.

Walter gives us a wakeup page at five minutes to six, and Lenny arrives minutes afterwards.

During morning rounds, Ken tells Lenny about our split-shift maneuver of last night where I came in to relieve him. Ken suggests that the three of us might want to do that for each other every night to avoid long periods without sleep.

"Set the alarm for two o'clock in the morning?" Lenny says. "Are you crazy? You guys can do that if you want to, but I need my beauty sleep."

"It hasn't helped so far," Ken says.

Everyone laughs.

In the end, Ken and I agree that we will split call for each other if we need to, such as when one of us is sick or hasn't slept for several days. Lenny can fend for himself. We have two cases this morning, but there's a delay in getting started because the anesthesiologists have a departmental meeting that none of us had heard about. The three of us stand in the operating room, and not even the scrub nurse or the circulating nurse is here yet when Ken comes up with a crazy idea.

"We're always standing over the patients," he says. "I wonder what it looks like to them."

Before any of us can say another word, Ken lies down on the operating table, on his back, looking up, while Lenny and I adjust the blinding overhead surgical lamps. We hover over him with our scrubs, caps and masks on, as though we were about to make an incision. It must be unnerving because Ken doesn't last more than a few seconds before he's up with an uneasy look. Then Lenny and I take our turns. When I lie down, my eyes meet his. I feel powerless and not at all in control of what is happening to me. I suspect that every patient we operate on feels that way, at least until the anesthesia hits. I hope I can remember those feelings.

CHAPTER 17

AN ANEURYSM AND A VALVE

Monday morning, and I am ready for another week of it. Today we have a patient who requires replacement of his aortic valve. Mr. Grant is a sixty-seven year old gentleman who has had increasing fatigue, shortness of breath and decreased exercise tolerance. Pre-op tests performed by his cardiologists disclosed that he has an aneurysm of the ascending aorta, and also a leaking aortic valve.

I visit briefly with Mr. Grant in Pre-op Clinic. He is a retired Professor of Mechanical Engineering. Ironically, he has spent his career studying fatigue and mechanical failure of cylindrical structures. That is just what has occurred to his enlarging aneurysmal aorta. He is remarkably well-informed and is resolved to get on with the surgical repair.

Dr. Martinez joins us in clinic to discuss some decisions that must be made about the operation. "We can use either a prosthetic valve that is made of a plastic-like material or a specially prepared pig valve. The prosthetic valve requires life-long anticoagulation, first with heparin, then with Coumadin—blood thinners, the non-medical public call them. But they don't really thin the blood; they just make it slower to clot. Alternatively, we could use a pig valve. This would not require anticoagulation, but pig valves last only 10 to 12 years and would require re-operation and replacement."

Mr. Grant went to the library where he studied the medical literature, and made a decision before he ever came to the hospital.

"I'm going to go with the prosthetic valve," he says. "I figure the joys of having your chest opened are probably overrated. "I'm not crazy about going through it once, let alone a second time."

I am pleased to deal with a well-informed patient.

Dr. Martinez, Paul and I take Mr. Grant to the operating room and begin the now familiar steps of cardio-thoracic surgery. Dr. Martinez replaces a portion of Mr. Grant's aorta with a Dacron graft, a cylindrical segment of Dacron with an artificial valve already sewn into it. This corrects his distended aorta, as well as his over-stretched aortic valve.

What makes the operation especially unusual is that his coronary arteries have to be cut off from his native aorta. Then they must be reattached to the new segment of Dacron aorta so they will supply blood to his heart. Dr. Martinez and Paul do the case. I help and watch with fascination as they cut little circular windows in the Dacron graft, and sew the delicate coronary arteries to the graft. They carefully align the vessels so that the coronaries don't twist or kink.

Fortunately, the replacement of the aorta and valve, and re-implantation of the coronary arteries goes well, and Mr. Grant is in the ICU by one o'clock. Dr. Martinez and I stand beside his bed discussing management of his fluids. His central line pressure measurements tell us that he has lots of fluid in his body, yet he's making only small amounts of urine. We adjust how much IV fluid we give him, and then we try to increase his urine output by using intravenous medications. We have to be careful not to let the potassium or sodium in his blood get too high or too low. Hey, this is fun—I feel like an internist; I'm getting to play doctor as well as plumber.

In the midst of all this decision-making, I receive a page from Edna in medical records.

"You're falling further behind on your undictated charts," she warns. "You're up to 22 now."

Undictated. Is there really such a word? If a chart has not been dictated in the first place, how can it be undictated? Can a scrambled egg be unscrambled? I know what she means; of course, but what can I say? I guess I'll have to use my spare time more wisely.

"It's a matter of priorities," I tell her. "Patient care comes before-eating, eating comes before sleeping, and sleeping comes before discharge summaries."

"Very clever," she says. "Do what you have to do, but I warn you. My supervisor won't stand for twenty undictated charts. He'll call the Chief of Staff's Office and they'll put a hold on your paycheck."

"I'll see what I can do."

***

Our second case today is William Nye, a sixty-seven year old gentleman with child-onset diabetes and terrible coronary artery disease. According to the cath lab findings, he's going to require a quadruple coronary artery bypass. Dr. McCarthy does the procedure faster than I could ever imagine. But, at the end of the operation, we can't get Mr. Nye off the bypass pump. His heart simply does not have the pumping strength. Dr. McCarthy tries again and again to shift the pumping load from the bypass machine to Mr. Nye's heart. But his ventricle is weak, and it cannot summon the pumping power.

But there is a device that we can use that often works quite well—an intra-aortic balloon pump. Walter prepares a sterile area in Mr. Nye's groin; we introduce a catheter into his femoral artery and advance it into his aorta. The system then works as follows: attached to the catheter is a thin-walled balloon. It is rapidly filled and emptied by an external pump. When Mr. Nye's heart relaxes and is not ejecting blood into his aorta, the pump rapidly fills the balloon, acting like an auxiliary heart. Conversely, when Mr. Nye's heart is contracting and pumping blood into his aorta, the system rapidly empties the balloon. This decreases the resistance against which his heart must pump. The external pump is timed by Mr. Nye's own EKG to fill and empty the balloon at precisely the right moments.

Thus, the balloon pump acts as a temporary auxiliary heart, giving Mr. Nye's heart a chance to regain its strength and pumping power. To avoid infection and injury to the blood cells, the balloon pump cannot remain in the aorta for more than three or four days, but often that is all that is required. Dr. McCarthy speaks of improvements in the balloon pump that may permit much longer durations of implantation.

In the operating room, the intra-aortic balloon pump proves to be effective in supporting Mr. Nye's heart. Dr. McCarthy and Paul complete the operation. Then we slide Mr. Nye off the operating table and onto a bed. As we wheel Mr. Nye into the ICU, Paul and I roll the refrigerator-size balloon pump console alongside his bed. For the next few days this clumsy piece of equipment will be his heart's best friend.

After Mr. Nye is stabilized in the ICU, I take the medical students out to Three East to examine the patients and see who might be ready for discharge. While the students load up the wheeled cart, I receive another page from Edna.

"Where are you?" she asks. "We need to talk."

Here comes trouble. "I'm on Three East. You can't miss me. I'm the mother hen with all the chicks."

"I'll be right up."

***

Although I've never seen her before, I can spot Edna the moment she steps off the elevator—gray-streaked, wiry brown hair pulled back in a librarian's bun, a tweed skirt that looks like it is woven of asbestos. There is something undeniably unattractive about her. Perhaps it's her bossy administrator's personality. She marches down the hall with unmistakable determination, fists clenched, and arms swinging side-to-side in front of her, like an iron curtain soldier on parade.

Offense is the best defense. "Edna, I'll get to those discharge summaries just as soon as I get some sleep."

"I understand," she says. "This isn't about medical records. I want to talk to you about Mr. Nye. He's my uncle. Tell me, how is he doing?"

"Well, you know I'm not supposed to give out information about patients except to the immediate family." I'm going to give her a dose of her own rules and regulations.

"But I am immediate family. He's my mother's brother, William Nye, William Stanley Nye."

"Well, I'm not sure..."

"It's okay. Really, it is. He's my uncle. He has diabetes, heart disease and some kidney problems."

She does seem to know him. Besides, as a person who works in the Medical Records Department, she has access to all the information in all the charts anytime she wants it.

"Well," I say. "I can tell you that today's operation went okay, but his heart isn't very strong, and we couldn't get him off the bypass pump. We had to put in a balloon pump. We'll see if we can wean him off that in the next few days."

"And if you can't?"

"Then he has to have a heart transplant."

"Or?"

"There is no or."

Edna listens attentively and seems to comprehend everything I say. "He's sixty-seven with a lot of medical problems," she says. "I'm not sure he'd be a candidate for a transplant."

"You may be right, but let's just wait and see."

She shrugs a little. "I appreciate your honesty." She starts to leave, then turns back to face me. "I'm sorry to keep harassing you about the incomplete medical records. It's my job."

"I understand. You do your job, and I'll do mine."

***

The ICU and the floor are both quiet and our team finishes rounds earlier than expected. We are sitting in the nurses' break room in the surgical ICU relaxing for a few minutes, too tired to face the automobile traffic humming outside the hospital. We are all surprised when Dr. Abraira, still dressed in scrubs, comes marching into the ICU with a large manila envelope crammed with chest films. They are from Mr. Haskins, a patient on whom Dr. McCarthy and Ken did a triple bypass. McCarthy is out of town with his family, and Dr. Abraira is covering all his professional responsibilities.

"Look at this," Dr. Abraira says. "These are Haskins' films, Albert Haskins, Dr. McCarthy's patient. Have you fellows been following him, regularly reviewing his films?"

We murmur a blended "yes."

Dr. Abraira selects a few films, and puts several of them up on the wall-mounted view box.

"Well, you all missed something important. In fact, even the radiologists missed it, at least until today when Dr. Vasquez spotted it. We can see by the presence of the chest tubes that these are post-op films." He points to a spot on each film. "Look here, what do you see?"

As my eyes accommodate to the reduced light of the view box, I can see a small, curved stainless steel surgical needle that must have been dropped into the chest cavity. It is about as small as a cut fingernail. With all the activity going on during a case, it is no surprise that such a small needle might have been dropped unnoticed. But it should have shown up in the needle count done by the nurses at the end of the case.

"I checked the nurse's report of operation form," Dr. Abraira says. "And they missed the count too, so there's plenty of blame to go around."

Thank goodness I didn't scrub on that case.

"Well," Dr. Abraira says. "A couple of days ago I went up to the third floor to see Mr. Haskins, and I told him about the missing needle. I explained that it is safe where it is isolated by soft tissue behind the heart. Mr. Haskins seemed to accept that explanation. That was a few days ago. But, when I saw him today, he said he spoke with a family member who is a physician, and I suspect he also spoke with a lawyer."

"Wouldn't you know it," Ken says under his breath.

"Haskins says he wants us to re-operate and take it out!"

"Really," Lenny says with surprise. "Who in the world would opt to have a repeat open chest operation when he really didn't need it?

Dr. Abraira continues. "I told him that x-rays show us approximately where the needle is, but it would be a major operation to actually find it. I explained that we would have to deal with the post-op adhesions, and the repeated surgery may increase the risk of developing an infection. The needle is probably concealed in loose soft tissue, or trapped and concealed by post-op adhesions so no matter how we try, we may not be able to find it. Although I didn't mention it to him, it's also a risk for us because we might easily be stuck by the needle increasing our risk of contracting hepatitis. But he insists that he wants it out because he's afraid the needle will get into the venous system and be carried by the flow stream into the heart. I hate to admit it, but it does sound possible."

"I don't know who he's been talking to," Paul says.

"Sure you do," Lenny says. "It sounds like someone who demands a re-operation, then sues for having to undergo it."

Dr. McCarthy calls every day to inquire as to the status of his patients. But he is especially concerned about Mr. Haskins. With every call, he offers to interrupt his trip and return to University Hospital.

Dr Abraira says, "No, I will take care of it."

On Tuesday afternoon, Dr. Abraira asks the residents, "Who of you might be willing to scrub on this case?"

None of us is eager to do so, but all of us agree that we will scrub if we are needed.

Abraira does the case with assistance from Walter. They operate calmly and deliberately, picking their way through post-op thoracic adhesions. Fortunately, no one is injured by the frustrating exercise. I'm curious to know if there are any legal issues as a result, but I do not have the nerve to ask. According to the statute of limitations, the operating team is legally liable for about two years. After some searching, they find the missing needle in a pillow of soft tissue.

CHAPTER 18

A VISIT FROM SANTA

Tonight is Christmas Eve. I call home to let my wife know that I'm on my way. "We have no cases scheduled for tomorrow," I tell her. "And I'm not on call; Lenny is. So, if everything goes well, I should be able to get out of here in just a few minutes."

"Great," my wife says. "The kids will be waiting up for you. When you come in through the garage, look in the trunk of my car; you'll find a bunch of gift-wrapped presents that Santa Claus left for you to give to the kids."

I walk to the locker room to change my clothes. I'm kind of curious. I wonder what Santa gave my kids for Christmas. I hope they are sensible gifts. I know what Santa gave me—not having to operate on Mr. Haskins to search for a lost needle, and a day off without having to be on call.

CHAPTER 19

INTEROFFICE MEMO

FROM: Chief of Staff
TO: Medical and surgical residents listed below:
Ken Wharton, M.D.
Philip Dobrin, M.D.
Robert Thompson, M.D.
Arthur Livitz, M.D.
SUBJECT: Incomplete Medical Records.
Pursuant to hospital policy regarding completion of incomplete medical records and, in accordance with hospital Bylaws (Article VII, section B), residents who have more than twenty-five undictated Discharge Summaries or have more than twenty-five incomplete medical records shall have their paychecks withheld until such time as their medical record deficiencies have been corrected.
CC: Chief of Medicine
     Chief of Surgery
     Marvin Smith, Payroll Office
     Edna Harmon, Medical Records Department

There I am on the list, right after Ken Wharton.

Tonight is our last night on the Cardiothoracic Surgery service. After we finish evening rounds, Ken and I go to Medical Records to pull out a couple of charts that contain our transcribed discharge summaries. Most of them are a page and a half or two pages long, and they have a lot of information about the patients: dates of admission and discharge, primary and secondary diagnoses, symptoms at the time of admission, cath lab results, surgical procedures performed, post-op course, complications, and status at the time of discharge. They also have lab results at the time of admission and discharge, X-ray reports, and other information that they don't really have to have, but seems essential to those of us who cared for them.

Then we look at one of Lenny Goldstein's discharge summaries. It's one short paragraph, and it contains only what is essential about the patient. Then we look at five of Lenny's discharge summaries. They're all the same, word for word. He must have dictated them from a single handwritten note card, a kind of recipe. Only the location of the blockages and the exact locations of the bypasses are different from patient to patient. He also lists complications, if there were any. Everything that is needed is right there. No wonder he's so up-to-date.

And why not? Discharge summaries are a paperwork exercise imposed by the insurance companies and the hospital accrediting agencies. Anyone who really wants to know about a patient's medical status is going to have to read the chart.

"I'll have my charts done in a week," I tell Ken.

"Me too."

That Lenny—always a star.

***

Ken, Lenny and I return to the ICU where Drs. Abraira, McCarthy and Martinez wait for us. The three white-coated attendings stand side-by-side like porcelain figures. Dr. Abraira looks each of us in the eye as he reaches out to shake our hands.

"Fellows, you did a fine job and I hope you learned a few things." His voice is calm and mellifluous.

"Oh, yes," I say. "We learned a lot."

"Good," Dr. Abraira says. " Now, I wish each of you good luck." Then the three attendings turn and start down the stairs to visit the cath lab. Tomorrow will bring three new residents who will face their own set of challenges.

"By the way," I ask. "Who is on tonight?"

"I am," Lenny says. "Everybody's stable, and I plan to keep it that way."

Knowing Lenny, I'm sure he will.

CHAPTER 20

BURNS AND PLASTIC SURGERY

I'm on my way to the Burn Unit to begin a new three-month rotation on Burns and Plastic Surgery. It sounds like a strange combination to me, but apparently it's not; a great deal of surgery is required immediately after an acute burn, and over time as it heals. In some patients, reconstructive procedures go on for years after an acute burn injury.

Lenny Goldstein will be on Burns and Plastics with me. We were on Cardiac Surgery together, and I am pleased with how well we got along, sharing the workload and keeping the rafts of data flowing.

Dr. Stanley Wisniewski is the Chief of Plastic Surgery. He arrives at the Burn Unit at about 6:40 a.m., brimming with energy and good humor. He is short with a giant walrus-like moustache and riveting black eyes. He is balding and, when he catches me sneaking a peek at his shiny pate, he flashes a big grin. "I part it in the middle; it's convenient, but it gives me a wide part."

At 6:45, Sheldon Ross, the Plastic Surgery Fellow, walks up to join our group. It seems rather nervy of him to show up for rounds after the attending has already been there and waiting. If I were to try that with Dr. Peterson, I would be in big trouble, but Dr. Wisniewski doesn't seem to care.

Sheldon is dressed casually in a long-sleeved, button-down, red checkered shirt with no tie or white lab coat. Here in the hospital, he doesn't look at all like a doctor.

"Good morning, Boss," Sheldon says as he walks up to Dr. Wisniewski. "Hi, guys," he says to Lenny and me without even turning to face us.

Yes, this fellow is quite informal.

Dr. Wisniewski glances down the corridor to the rooms housing burned patients. "Right now we have four active burn patients and four cosmetic surgery patients. Let's see how they are doing." We walk down the hall to a group of rooms designated by a wall plaque as Burn Unit. Family Members Only. We don gloves, caps and yellow disposable paper gowns that are clean, but not sterile.

"In some hospitals," Wisniewski says. "Burned patients are managed by a doctor who is solely dedicated to burn care, a so-called burnologist. In this hospital, we plastic surgeons take care of the burned patients. It makes sense for us since we do so much skin grafting and reconstructive surgery during and after the burn has healed."

We stop at the first patient's room. It contains just one bed in the center of the room with a ventilator sitting beside it. Stainless steel tables are lined up along one wall where they are stacked three feet high with packs of sterile gauze and plastic bottles of iodine-containing antibacterial solutions. This iodine-rich solution gives off an astringent medicinal odor that permeates the room and every crevice and pore.

The patient, swaddled in disinfectant-soaked gauze, is festooned with IV's in his arms, a feeding tube in his nose, an endotracheal tube connected to the ventilator and an assortment of bedside pumps that regulate his IV fluids. He also has a latex catheter in his urinary bladder that drains dark golden urine into a plastic bag that hangs at the side of the bed. Dr. Wisniewski introduces us to the patient.

"This is Rodney Jackson. He's a 30 year-old man who was transferring gasoline from one car to another. Evidently, no one reminded him to discard his glowing cigarette before he poured the gas. Rodney has a thirty percent of body surface area burn of his arms, face and neck. And he has another problem; the fire burned his airway, an inhalation injury. For now, he's on a ventilator."

We return to the hall where Lenny asks Dr. Wisniewski about the patient's prognosis.

"We expect him to survive," Wisniewski says. "But he'll require numerous skin grafts to replace the full thickness burns on his arms, face and neck. Mortality increases markedly in patients who have more than 40 percent burns. But first, there's the question of whether his airway will recover enough for him to be able to breathe on his own. Right now, he's dependent on the ventilator."

I scribble Wisniewski's survival statistics on a three-by-five card.

"Let's face it," he says. "A serious burn is just about the worst injury a person can sustain. And the larger the burn, the greater the mortality. Especially in kids and the elderly." He glances at his watch as if to gauge how much longer he can remain with us.

"Treating these patients is a challenge," he says. "First, they lose a lot of fluid through the burn, so prompt fluid replacement is essential. We give them lots of fluid through the IV—two, three times normal requirements, with half given in the first eight hours. Sheldon will go over the formulas we use to estimate target volumes, but those are just estimates." He turns to Lenny. "Tell us; how do we know that we are giving a patient enough IV fluid?"

"By tracking the urine output."

"Right. And remember: Early replacement makes all the difference. Once you get behind, you may never be able to catch up. So we give half of the computed requirement in the first eight hours. But you have to be careful in the elderly that you don't throw them into heart failure.

"Another thing to remember is that the patients lose protein as they leak fluid out through the wound. We can give them intravenous protein, but it's controversial, especially early in the treatment. It tends to leak out of the blood vessels, taking water with it, causing the tissues to swell.

"By the way," Wisniewski says. "We're a regional burn center. Doctors at other hospitals call wanting to transfer burned patients to us. We're glad to take them if we have a bed. But be sure the patient they want to send has a large bore IV, and has received plenty of fluid. Sometimes outside physicians are so eager to get a patient out of their ER that they lie about how much fluid the patient's received. We've reported a couple of outside hospitals to the county for inappropriate transfers."

Dr. Wisniewski falls silent for a moment as he again checks his watch. "Now, let's talk about wound care. We cover the burn with gauze impregnated with iodine-containing Betadine. A lot of burn units prefer silver sulfadiazine. They're both antibacterial. When the eschar—the leathery burned skin—begins to separate from the living tissue beneath it, we surgically remove the eschar. That reduces the risk of infection in that dead tissue that's just sitting there."

"Whacking off the dead stuff," Sheldon mutters. "Not exactly precision surgery."

"No, it's not," Wisniewski says. "But it needs to be done. It can be messy. The patients usually lose a lot of blood. Nowadays we're pretty aggressive about it, and we do early skin grafting to protect the wound.

"In a burn unit, the nurses and the nursing assistants do a lot of the work, changing the dressings every six to eight hours, debriding the eschar as it loosens."

"What about antibiotics?" Lenny asks.

"We give all the patients tetanus boosters and frequent doses of pain medication, but we give antibiotics only when we see clear evidence of infection, and we have cultured the organism."

Sheldon puts his hands in his pockets and impatiently jingles loose change.

"We don't want to encourage the development of bacterial resistance in the Burn Unit if we can help it." Sheldon says.

"One more principle," he adds. "It's important to maintain nutrition, by mouth or by threading a nasogastric tube through the patient's nose and into the stomach, or even by intravenous feedings.

"The burn makes the patients hypermetabolic. They burn calories at a phenomenal rate. And they need a lot of protein to heal and cope with infection. Plus, of course, we have to make up for the protein they lose weeping through the burned skin."

Dr. Wisniewski checks his watch again. "Hey, I'm late. I have a meeting with the dean. Sheldon will stay here, and finish up with you." And as quickly as he arrived, Dr. Wisniewski leaves—moustache, wide part, and all.

Sheldon steps forward to take over rounds. "Look, I'll help you guys whenever you need it, but you are going to run the Burn Unit, not me. I'm really not interested in taking care of acutely sick people anymore. I did five years of General Surgery. Now I'm in my last two years of Plastics. That's enough. My real interest is in cosmetic surgery—boobs, noses, facelifts. Preferably in California. That's where the money is."

As usual, Lenny hasn't said much, and I wonder what his opinions are of Sheldon's career plans. I'm not sure that I know what I think of them myself. After seven years of training, Sheldon is entitled to get on with his life, and I'm sure he has an impatient wife at home who reminds him of that every day.

Sheldon writes orders in Mr. Jackson's chart—IV fluids, intravenous nutrition and ventilator settings. "Anesthesia will be up in a little while to adjust the ventilator, if they think it needs adjustment."

Before we leave Mr. Jackson, Sheldon promises that he will explain the choice and quantity of IV fluids that he's ordered. "There's a lot of detail concerning the composition of the fluids" he adds. "And we'll discuss it later"

Lenny's got that omniscient look that tells me he read it all before he got here.

Our second patient is Stanley Borowski, a 40 year-old electrician. He was working on a high-tension tower when he took a nearly fatal electrical shock. He is lucky not to have been thrown off the tower and broken his neck.

"He's been in the coronary ICU," Sheldon says. "These electrical burns can cause serious injuries to the cardiac conducting system. Sometimes they develop arrhythmias that don't show up for weeks.

"The burns are on his hands. They're just a small percentage of body surface area, but if you lose the function of your palms and fingers, you're in big trouble."

The three of us file into Mr. Borowski's room, and Sheldon introduces us to the patient.

Mr. Borowski gives us a big smile, apparently glad to have some company. "I'd shake your hands, but you don't want to grab these paws." His hands are wrapped in bulky gauze and are as large as catcher's mitts. Then he turns to Sheldon. "Hey, Doc, when am I going to get out of here?"

"I've told you every day for the past week, Mr. Borowski. As soon as we get your hands fixed up. Besides, that heart monitor you're connected to is your pal. You can't go anywhere without it for a few more days—whatever the cardiologists tell us. They're in charge of your heart problems."

"I didn't know I had heart problems."

"You don't," Sheldon snaps. "At least, not yet. I've told you that again and again."

When we leave Mr. Borowski, Sheldon turns to us. "I've told him a half dozen times about the heart rhythm business. He just can't seem to get it. I guess a couple thousand volts will do that to you."

"Okay," Lenny says. "He's confused after being zapped with a thousand volts. But that's not his fault. Give the guy a break."

"I suppose," Sheldon says.

Our third patient is LeShauna Orlean, a one year-old child with symmetric burns from her toes to high up on her thighs. She's lying in a crib sobbing inconsolably as one of the nurses rubs her back. Another nurse stands at the sink preparing her bottle.

Pediatrics and the Burn Service are jointly caring for this child," Sheldon says. "These burns are highly suspicious," one of the nurses says. "They look deliberate in such a small child who is too young to climb up and step with both feet into a hot tub, and then climb out. Anyway, who makes a scalding hot bath for a one year old child? We think the mother or her boyfriend got tired of listening to the kid bawl. In fact, she was brought into the Emergency Room with a small burn on her arm three months ago."

Sheldon points to a two-inch-long scar on the child's upper arm. "The authorities are looking into it."

"Bastards," Lenny mutters, shaking his head. "How could anyone do that to a kid, or to anybody? It's criminal."

It's the first time I've seen Lenny so upset.

We return to Mr. Jackson, our first patient, to inspect his now-exposed gasoline fire wounds. The Burn Unit nurses give him a preparatory dose of narcotic. Then they gown and glove, and remove the Betadine-soaked bandages wrapped around his arms, neck and hands. They move slowly, inch by inch, gently handling the traumatized areas. Still, Mr. Jackson cries out and withdraws with every touch. We examine each wound and note the eschar. It is the hardening burnt skin that is separating from the underlying wound. From Mr. Jackson's responses, it appears that some of the wounds are partial thickness and innervated as they are unbearably painful, even after the administration of narcotics.

"It's like this," Sheldon says. "The wounds are less painful where the burn is full thickness, and has destroyed the skin and nerves. Mr. Jackson's pain response to the nurses' debridement tells us that at least some of his wounds are partial thickness and remain innervated."

The regions not covered by skin are disturbing to see, raw flesh with tendons and blood vessels. It reminds me of a dissected cadaver in Anatomy class.

"We'll be able to graft some of these Crispy Critters pretty soon," Sheldon says.

"Crispy Critters!" Lenny repeats. He looks at Sheldon with disbelief. "These burn wounds are intensely painful, and disfiguring for life. Even if only joking, how could anyone..."

"It's just an expression some of the residents use," Sheldon says, shrugging a little.

But Lenny will have none of it. He shakes his head with disapproval.

After we write notes describing the burned sites and the patients' overall condition, we leave the Burn ICU. We remove our caps, gloves, gowns and booties at the door. Then we wash our hands, put on fresh scrubs, and walk out to see the Plastic Surgery patients on the floor who had undergone cosmetic surgery.

***

Sheldon speaks with each patient who had undergone cosmetic surgery, asking them about their discomfort. Then he removes their bandages so we can inspect their wounds. There are four patients, each having undergone a procedure to enhance their appearance. One woman had breast implants, one had surgery to reduce the size of her nose, a third patient was a young man who had surgery to alter the appearance of his chin, a fourth patient is a middle-aged woman who underwent a facelift to make her look younger. This was her second facelift over a 10 or 12 year period.

It strikes me that our dualistic service, Burns and Plastic Surgery, treats some of the most and least severely injured patients in the hospital. And, unlike the burned patients, those admitted for cosmetic surgery are here by choice, rather than misfortune. We write notes and orders in the charts, and discharge all four patients

150

to return to clinic in three days. Then we head to the operating room for today's cases.

"There's going to come a time," Sheldon says, "when we'll do all these cosmetic procedures on an outpatient basis. We'll give them anesthesia, do the procedure, and then recover them from anesthesia. When they're fully awake, we'll send them home. There's a lot of financial pressure to do so, and it will be here sooner than you think."

Back when I was with Barney on General Surgery, he made the same prediction. We seem to be moving to an outpatient model of care, rather than an inpatient model. And it might not be a bad idea, as there's lots of data showing that hospitals are a reservoir of infection. Of course, those patients who require sophisticated complex technologies may still require inpatient services. We're not going to be doing brain surgery on the patient's kitchen table.

"But for now," Sheldon says. "You guys have the job of writing up the Histories and Physicals for each surgery, and dictating each Discharge Summary. We have several a day, so keep up with them. If the History and Physical is not in the chart before surgery, the OR nurses won't let the case begin."

There's no escaping the paperwork.

Lenny and I change into fresh scrubs, then we enter the OR to watch Dr. Wisniewski and Sheldon perform a facelift on a fifty year old woman. It's fascinating to watch them free the skin from the underlying bone, then pull the skin up toward the ears to tighten it, smoothing out the wrinkles. I notice that, although Sheldon is highly skilled and has seven years of surgical experience, he mainly assists Dr. Wisniewski, and does little of the case himself. Of course, at this stage of his career, Sheldon has all the requisite technical skills; what he is learning is what to do and when to do it, not how to do it. Therefore, he learns a great deal by assisting and observing.

The patients have come to Dr. Wisniewski because they want the skills and training of an expert Plastic

Surgeon. Thus, there is a tug between providing the patient with the experienced attending versus training of the fellow. The resolution seems to be a gradual increase in the participation by the trainee under the close supervision of the attending. Dr. Wisniewski promises Lenny and me that we'll get to scrub and help on some of the cases, but I don't expect to be doing anything complex.

After the scheduled cosmetic cases have been completed, Wisniewski, Sheldon, Lenny and I return to the Burn ICU to examine the burn patients after the dressings have been removed.

Dr. Wisniewski stares down at the raw gasoline-burned arms of Mr. Jackson. "It's time to take the eschar off," he says. "Better get the family to sign a surgical consent for him, and type and cross him for two units of blood. We have a light schedule tomorrow. Maybe the OR will let us fit him in."

***

Lenny and I start morning rounds at 6:30. We begin in the Burn Unit where we gown and glove, inspect each patient's wounds, and write orders and notes in the charts. Then we remove our clean paper garb, and head out of the Burn Unit to see the patients on the floor who underwent cosmetic surgery yesterday.

First, we see Mrs. Clowes, the fifty year old lady who had a facelift yesterday. "This is my second one," she says. "The first time was about ten years ago."

I carefully unwrap her bandages. Her face is severely discolored from bleeding under the skin. One eye is swollen.

"Ow-ow-ow!" she cries out as I undo the gauze.

According to protocol she should be discharged today. "Do you have someone at home who can help you for the next few days?" I ask.

"My husband. He'll be coming to pick me up this morning."

I write a prescription for pain medication, and give her an appointment to Plastic Surgery clinic. I gaze at her battered face again. To look forever young. Is it worth it? I guess it must be in our appearance-conscious world. It seems analogous to the pain of giving birth; women tend to forget the pain of delivery over time as they delight in the outcome. Of course, they become pregnant with the second and third child before the first one blossoms into an unrewarding teenager.

The next patient is Mr. Bright, a man in his early twenties who underwent insertion of a prosthesis to enlarge his small chin. Our meeting with him is a quick examination of his post-op wound, a prescription for pain which he rejects, a note and an order in the chart: "Home today. Return to clinic in three days."

Sheldon, are you sure you want to do this for the rest of your professional life? I muse to myself,

After we finish on the floor, Lenny and I head to the cafeteria for breakfast. Lenny doesn't have much to say.

"How do you like Plastics?" I ask him.

"It's okay, but we haven't seen much of it yet."

"Maybe this is all there is."

"Could be," he says with a noncommittal shrug.

We're sitting quietly when Sheldon pages us. "Come to the OR. We are about to begin our first case."

By the time we get there, change our clothes and scrub, Rodney Jackson is already asleep under the protective eye of Dr. Hakeem. Dr. Wisniewski and Sheldon are carving off the eschar, scrambling to get clamps and small ligatures on the vessels connecting the eschar to the underlying tissues.

Sheldon was right—this is a blood bath. In fact, the sterile drapes on the patient are slick with blood. Dr. Wisniewski controls those vessels that are too small to be clamped with the electrocautery. Lenny and I pitch in, clamping and cauterizing as fast as we can in order to keep from losing too much blood. Out of the corner of my eye I can see Dr. Hakeem infusing blood intravenously, trying to match our losses.

After we get the bleeding under control, we focus on the patients' thighs where Dr. Wisniewski and Sheldon use a hand-held pneumatically-driven device that looks like an electric beard trimmer. This device is used to excise a thin sheet of skin, a skin graft. I watch Sheldon apply grafts to the bare wounds on Mr. Jackson's arms. Then he places stitches along the edges of the grafts to hold them in place. Finally, I get the opportunity to apply a skin graft with Sheldon guiding and directing me. I place each anchoring stitch with as much care and precision as I can muster. Lenny is doing the same.

"Don't waste a centimeter of that skin," Dr. Wisniewski cautions. "These grafts are precious. They will help prevent the wound shrinkage and the terrible contractures that occur when burns heal on their own."

As we finish, I look down at the operative field. Mr. Jackson's arms look like a patchwork quilt, a farmer's field viewed from low altitude. Sheldon is right. This isn't very elegant surgery, but it certainly is more gratifying than fixing noses and doing breast implants in women who are eager to charm that certain someone they see in the mirror.

When we've done all that we can for today, we transfer Mr. Jackson to a gurney, and return him to his room in the Burn unit. After we get Mr. Jackson settled, we stop to talk with Rita, the head nurse on the burn unit. She's a middle-aged lady with strong maternal instincts and lots of common sense.

"A lady from the county came by today to see the baby," she says. "She didn't say much, but she examined the child, and she looked very concerned. She took extensive notes and photographs. I told her that we hadn't seen the parents since they first brought the child in."

"Good," I say. "I'm glad someone's concerned about that kid. It sure looks like child abuse."

"It does indeed, and that child's going to be scarred forever."

"And, oh by the way." Rita adds. "We have a new patient, a Mr. Martensen, burned in a chemical fire. Presumably, it's a 40 percent body surface area burn to his arms and trunk, but we haven't taken the gauze wraps off yet."

"Anyway, the other hospital told us they put in an IV and gave him three liters (3,000 cc) of fluid, but wait till you see this." She leads us into Mr. Martensen's room. The patient is sitting upright in bed swathed in gauze with a modest blue Butterfly IV in his arm through which he's received a mere 300 or 400 cc of fluid, a far cry from the claimed 3,000 cc. The IV bag hanging beside him is still half full. He has a Foley catheter in his urinary bladder with just a small amount of dark, highly concentrated urine in the collection bag. This man needs much more IV fluid, as fast as we get it into him.

"Can you imagine sending us a patient like this," Rita says. "It's positively criminal." She shakes her head in disbelief.

Rita and her team of nurses gown and glove, and begin to remove Mr. Martensen's bandages while Lenny and I prepare to draw blood, and start intravenous lines to provide substantial amounts of IV fluid.

***

It's seven-thirty in the evening, and Lenny and I are eager to leave for the night. It's been a long day, but before we go, we must take care of all the elective admissions scheduled for tomorrow's cosmetic surgery cases. Harriet, one of my favorite night nurses, tells me that we have one last admission for plastic surgery, on her floor, a Miss Sanders.

"She's late getting here," Harriet says. "But she's the last one."

I find a clipboard and head down the hall to admit her.

According to the Admission Form, she's a 22 year-old woman here for "Revision of breast implants." I stop before I enter her room, and wave to Harriet. "Come along, Harriet," I say. "I need you in there. It's not a good idea for a male doctor to see a female patient without a nurse in the room."

When we enter her room, we find Miss Sanders sitting on the edge of her bed dressed only in a cotton hospital gown. She is unusually attractive, and I can only wonder why she thinks she needs cosmetic surgery, but that's up to her and her doctor, not me.

She has dark hair, and is made up as if waiting for her date to arrive to take her out for a night on the town.

She radiates the self-assurance of a woman one who has been admired all her life.

I pull up a chair beside her hospital bed, introduce myself, and ask my usual opening question—"What brings you to the hospital at this time?"

"Dr. Wisniewski did breast implants about a year ago," she says. "But I'd like him to make them larger. I saw him in clinic, and he said he could do it." She hesitates for a moment. "But maybe they're okay the way they are. I'll be interested to hear what you think of them."

"Frankly," I tell her, "it doesn't matter what I think. I'm just a resident here, filling out the paperwork for tomorrow's surgery. What you decide about surgery is between you and Doctor Wisniewski."

"I'm not asking you as a doctor," she insists. "I'm asking you as a man."

"Right now, I'm just a doctor." Out of the corner of my eye, I see Harriet covering her mouth, stifling a nervous laugh.

Miss Sanders has managed to put the flimsy cotton hospital gown on backwards so that it now opens in the front instead of in the back. In the midst of our conversation she hops off the bed, turns toward me and without hesitation or embarrassment opens her cotton gown. At that moment I find myself staring "nose-to-nose" at her emblems of womanhood.

"Well," she asks, "What do you think?"

I am caught in the crush of a dilemma, for anything I say will be the wrong thing. "Look," I say. "I'm only the resident, and my opinion doesn't count."

Miss Sanders is annoyed, but I stick to my guns.

I ask Harriet to stand close beside me so she can observe everything I do as I record Miss Sanders' medical history. Then I perform the requisite pre-operative physical examination. I obtain Miss Sanders' signature on the consent form for tomorrow's surgery, and then, just as fast as my feet will carry me I head for the nearest elsewhere. I do not know just where that is, but I do know it's not in Miss Sanders' room.

Harriet and I walk briskly down the hall together, stride for stride, staring straight ahead.

"So," Harriet asks. "What did you think?"

"Think about what?"

"About Miss Sanders."

"It doesn't matter what I think. That's up to her boyfriend or husband or Dr. Wisniewski, or just about anybody, but not me."

When we get back to the nurses' station, Lenny is sitting there, writing up the History and Physical for a middle-aged lady who is being admitted for a facelift. Lenny looks up at me, and I regale him with my tenuous adventures with Miss Sanders.

Lenny is not impressed. "Delusions of glandeur," he says with a disinterested shrug.

***

It's 7:30 in the morning. Lenny and I are in the Burn Unit making morning rounds. As usual, Sheldon is off somewhere doing who-knows-what. I'm writing IV orders for Mr. Jackson when my pager goes off directing me to call the OR Stat! I'm on the phone in a flash. It's Dr. Wisniewski, and I can tell from his tone that he is mightily upset.

"What did you tell Diane Sanders last night?" he asks

"Nothing. NOT A THING. Why? What did she say I said?"

"When we got her to the operating table, she sat up and said that she changed her mind. She said that the resident who saw her last night told her that her implants were fine and that she should leave them alone."

I'm feeling very much in trouble. "Not true," I say,. "Ask Harriet, the nurse. She was in the room with me, start to finish. The patient asked me what I thought of her implants, and I told her that was between her and her doctor and her boyfriend or husband. Otherwise I had no opinion."

There's a long and worrisome telephone pause. Then Wisniewski starts to laugh. "Well, don't worry about it. This is the second time she's changed her mind on the operating table. She's a kook. Next time she wants us to revise her implants; she can find someone else to do it."

Yes, I think to myself—she would be perfect for Sheldon.

CHAPTER 21

THE AIRWAY

Today I begin a three month rotation on the Anesthesiology Service, so I introduce myself to Dr. Hakeem, the Chief of Anesthesia. He invites me into his office and offers me a glass of sweet hot tea.

Dr. Hakeem's office is a portrait of chaos. The room is filled with stacks of unread journals, piles of Egyptian newspapers and a mishmash of reports awaiting his review and signature. This is a far cry from the stylish surgeons' offices that I have visited. On the desk in the center of the office is a round inch-thick glass ashtray choked with several weeks' worth of musty mashed cigarette butts. How, I wonder can an anesthesiologist, the keeper of the airway smoke cigarettes?

Dr. Hakeem greets me with a warm smile. He is bald with a pronounced monk's cap, a ring of frizzy black hair that peeks out above his ears and below his surgical cap. His rotund belly pushes out in front of him, straining against his scrubs, threatening to consume the edge of his beleaguered desk. "Welcome," he says with an unmistakable Arabic accent. "Have a seat. I am Dr. Hakeem, the Chief of Anesthesia." He reaches out to me with a warm handshake. "We knew from the schedule that you would be coming, and we have been looking forward to meeting you." He motions to a chair.

I take a seat...

"Let me tell you about anesthesia," he says. "It is applied pharmacology. We wish to prevent the patient from feeling pain, we want him not to move so the surgeons can do their operation, and we want him to have no memory of the procedure. We can do all those things with the drugs you learned about in medical school." He waves his hands. "We use them everyday in Anesthesiology, and you will learn to use them, too."

I nod in return. I suspect that every surgical resident who has ever walked through his doorway has heard Hakeem's proud spiel. Moreover, I suspect that Hakeem has harbored the hope that sooner or later, a surgical resident would switch his career from Surgery to Anesthesia—what greater approbation could there be than that? But I have never heard of it occurring, at least not in this university's Surgery and Anesthesia training programs.

Hakeem gathers his thoughts for a moment. "You surgeons," he says, wagging a disapproving finger. "Sometimes you abuse us and treat us like second-class citizens, but you can't operate without us." He flashes a sly smile. "You need us up there at the head of the table; above that towel we hang to separate us from the operation." He pauses again. "Do you know what we call it, that towel?"

"An ether screen?"

"Very good." Hakeem rolls his eyes in wonderment. "From the days when we used ether for anesthesia."

"Years ago," he continues, "When Dr. Blumenthal was operating here, he abused us something terrible. Shouting and complaining all the time. Nothing we did was good enough, even though his patients did well. It was all the time war. You know what I called the ether screen in those days, that towel that separated us from Blumenthal?"

Hakeem answers his own question. "The Gaza strip." He erupts into boisterous laughter, slapping his thigh. I suspect he has told that joke to a thousand captive ears, and that he has enjoyed it each time as much as he did the first time. "Blumenthal is gone," he says. "But we are still here."

"The surgeon should do his job," Hakeem says. "And he should leave us alone so we can do ours." He pulls his chair forward, its wooden feet scraping fitfully on the uneven floor. "What we do is important," he says. "Can you imagine doing surgery in the old days, before anesthesia? Or worse yet, can you imagine being the patient?"

The notion of performing surgery or being a patient without anesthesia is unthinkable.

Hakeem says. "Let me show you around." He rises from behind his desk and guides me to the locker room where I change quickly into scrubs. When I rejoin him, he leads me to a room just outside the operating rooms. A brass plate on the door reads Pre-Op Holding Area. It is a large space with a row of gurneys lined up along each wall. Some are waiting for a patient; others are occupied with a patient waiting to be to be transported to the operating room.

Each patient has an intravenous line in his arm to give him fluid before surgery, and to provide intravenous access for administering medications.

"This is Mr. Edlin," Hakeem says, pointing to a sleeping, gray-haired gentleman on a gurney. "Dr. Peterson is going to fix his hernia, and you will be the anesthesia resident on this case. But don't worry," he adds. "We will teach you what you need to know. You will see when you examine his medical history. He is a good first case for a beginning anesthesia resident like yourself. And, of course, Dr. Chung, a fully-trained anesthesiologist, will be present with you throughout the case."

I see from the chart that Mr. Edlin is a healthy 51-year old male who takes no medications and has no allergies. Dr. Chung will give him a spinal. It is very safe.

Hakeem gives Mr. Edlin a pat on the shoulder. "And we gave him a little Valium pre-op too, to make him calm. "Isn't that right, Mr. Edlin?"

But the Valium is doing its job, and Mr. Edlin snores soundly, deep in sleep. When Mr. Edlin is wheeled into the operating room, I walk beside him. There I meet Dr. Chung, an unusually tall, slender, black-haired Chinese gentleman with a perpetual smile. He extends his outstretched hand to me.

His speech is a mixture of mangled English and Americanized Chinese. I can't decipher more than a word or two here and there. He must know that he is difficult to understand because, as he speaks, he points and gesticulates like a conductor directing a symphony orchestra. He raises and lowers his voice too, as if to emphasize what he is saying. But none of it helps; I cannot understand more than a word or two of what he says. It supports my contention that the universal scientific language is not English; it is broken English.

After we transfer Mr. Edlin to the operating table, Dr. Hakeem joins us to help administer the spinal anesthesia. For this, we awaken Mr. Edlin and help him to sit with his feet dangling over the side of the operating table. Dr. Chung paints Mr. Edlin's back with pungent, dark brown iodine-containing disinfectant; then he uses a long thin needle to probe for an opening between the vertebrae through which he can pass the needle. Once through, he searches for the dural sac through which the spinal nerves pass.

When he is able to draw back spinal fluid through his long needle, he injects a carefully determined quantity of local anesthetic.

We quickly return Mr. Edlin to a supine position on the operating table. Repeatedly, we touch his skin lightly here and there with the point of a sharp needle to determine the level to which the anesthesia is effective. We want him to be numb well down to his legs.

We wait for the anesthesia to take full effect, tilting him slightly—first head up, and then head down—to distribute the anesthetic, and achieve just the right level of it. While waiting, we watch the EKG screen monitoring Mr. Edlin's heart rhythm. It is persistently normal.

After a few minutes, Dr. Peterson strides into the room trailing his platoon of surgical residents and students. "You guys done fooling around?" he asks.

"Just a minute more," Dr. Hakeem responds. "We want to be certain of the level of anesthesia"

Dr. Peterson scowls and stares at the wall clock.

"All right," Hakeem says. "Any time you are ready."

"We've been ready for the last half hour."

Dr. Chung turns to explain something to Dr. Peterson, but from the surgeon's bewildered expression, I can see that he does not understand a word of it any better than I do.

"It's like listening to wallpaper," Peterson says, shaking his head.

I wonder how Chung can function as an anesthesiologist when it is almost impossible to understand him. And is it safe for him to give anesthesia? How can he and his colleagues communicate with one another?

As though he could read my thoughts, Dr. Hakeem lowers his voice and speaks discreetly to me about Dr. Chung.

"It's hard for us to understand him, but he follows everything we say. We sent him to a speech therapist, a Chinese-American speech therapist at that. It didn't help one bit. But don't underestimate him. He's very skilled, and he scored very high on the written Board exams in Anesthesia."

All that may be true. But I still would have misgivings if Dr. Chung were giving anesthesia to a member of my family.

Dr. Peterson and his residents scrub at the sink outside the operating room, while we carefully monitor our sleeping patient. He has no sensation from the navel down. A few minutes later, the surgical team returns to the room to gown and glove. Then they drape Mr. Edlin, and make an incision in the groin. I watch as they identify a weak area in the abdominal wall, reduce the hernia sac to its proper domain in the abdomen, carefully place a mesh over a large abdominal wall defect, and sew it into place. Then they close the skin.

This is a novel perspective for me, observing a procedure that I know from hands-on surgical experience, but watching it now over the ether screen as a spectator. I have an indirect sense of participation. Is this how the anesthesiologists feel about all surgical cases—a part of the procedure, but kept at a distance by the ether screen?

Throughout the case, I monitor Mr. Edlin closely. Following Dr. Chung's and Dr. Hakeem's direction, I enter his pulse rate, blood pressure and respiratory rate on a preprinted form called an Anesthesia Flow Sheet. It's a simple task, tedious, really, as Mr. Edlin snores through the entire procedure.

After his hernia has been repaired and his skin has been closed, we awaken him, slide him onto a gurney, and wheel him into the Post Anesthesia Recovery Room where he will be under the watchful eye of the Recovery Room nurses. Their job is to monitor his pulse, blood pressure, respiratory rate and urine output. If there are any problems, they will call for one of the anesthesiologists to evaluate him.

While we are out of the operating room, the OR custodians prepare the room for the next case. They wash the thin plastic mats that serve as mattresses on the operating table, and talk among themselves in some eastern European language as they wet mop the floor. The stinging odor of disinfectant pervades the room.

Dr. Peterson hovers nearby. "You know," he says impatiently to Dr. Hakeem. "I've got better things to do than watch your guys learn how to give anesthesia and wet-mop the floor. Your turn-around-time between cases must be terrible."

Dr. Hakeem shrugs. He is just as much a professional as Dr. Peterson, and he administers anesthesia in a safe and judicious fashion. Washing the floor is not part of the anesthesiologist's job; it is the custodian's task. But it seems that Dr. Blumenthal's impatient spirit still roams the halls of these operating rooms.

According to my watch, the OR custodians have spent only eight minutes waiting for the wet floor to dry. But that's about all it takes to get Dr. Peterson fired up.

"We'll be ready as soon as the floor is dry," Hakeem says.

In the pre-op holding area, Dr. Hakeem introduces me to the next patient, Mrs. DeAngelo. "She is a forty-five year old lady with right upper quadrant abdominal pain. The pain appears after meals, especially after eating fatty foods. These symptoms are consistent with gall bladder disease, and a sonogram discloses that she does, indeed, have stones in the gall bladder. This morning, Dr. Peterson and his residents are going to remove her gall bladder with its contained stones."

Dr. Hakeem and I wheel her into the operating room. "This is a bigger operation than the hernia," he says. "And it's higher up on the abdomen, too high for spinal anesthesia. We'll put her to sleep."

We ask Mrs. DeAngelo to slide from the gurney onto the operating table. After Dr. Peterson greets her, we place a mask over her nose and mouth to provide oxygen. At the same time, Dr. Hakeem infuses a small amount of Valium and a narcotic through an IV in her arm. Then he adds an inhalation anesthetic in the mask to provide some additional pain control. He also infuses a small dose of a paralytic agent to relax the abdominal wall musculature. This will permit the surgeons to open and operate within her abdomen. Otherwise her abdominal muscles would be too tense to permit access.

"I tell you secret of anesthesia," Hakeem says. "Moderation. The drugs we use are effective when we use them separately, but some require high doses. And at high doses, they have side effects on the heart and respiration. But when we use several of them together, all in lower doses, they are effective and have fewer side effects. You see? Moderation."

"But now," Hakeem says, "I teach you the most useful skill you can learn while you're in Anesthesia—placing an endotracheal tube in the trachea to maintain an airway. It can be lifesaving." He hands me a steel, L-shaped device about the size of my hand. It's called a laryngoscope, and it has a tiny battery-operated light in the arm of the L that is inserted into the mouth and throat.

Dr. Hakeem advances the device until it reaches to the back of Mrs. DeAngelo's throat. "Have a look," he says.

I look, but see nothing; the oral cavity is obscured by saliva.

Hakeem uses a suction tube to dry the mouth and throat. Then I'm able to see the pink moist mucosa that forms the inner lining of her mouth and throat.

Dr. Hakeem motions to me to take the apparatus. "Now lift her tongue with the laryngoscope," Hakeem says. "And make sure you can see the epiglottis where it guards the entrance to the airway. You have to lift it out of the way."

I do as instructed. Mrs. DeAngelo is lying on her back, and her tongue tends to fall back and into her throat. In order to be able to see, and to prevent her tongue from blocking her airway, I use the laryngoscope to push her tongue and epiglottis aside. This reveals her vocal cords and airway leading into her trachea and lungs.

"You must see the vocal cords where they frame the entrance to the trachea," Hakeem says. "It's one of the best ways to be sure you're in the airway." Then he hands me a curved plastic tube called an endotracheal tube.

"This is to put in the trachea to provide an airway," Hakeem says. "But first, hold the laryngoscope with your left hand. This will help you hold the tongue to one side while you identify the epiglottis and the cords. Then use your right hand to advance the endotracheal tube."

It sounds simple enough—use the left hand to push the tongue to the left and, while doing that, advance the plastic endotracheal tube into the airway. But it's not so easy because the tongue repeatedly escapes the restraint provided by the laryngoscope. Nevertheless, I identify the landmarks and insert the endotracheal tube.

Once I am in what I think is the trachea, Dr. Hakeem attaches a brown plastic football-like bag to the outer end of the endotracheal tube that I just inserted. He calls it an Ambu bag, and he squeezes the bag rhythmically to deliver oxygen into the lungs. "Now," he says. "Take a stethoscope and listen to be sure the tube is in the trachea, and not in the esophagus and stomach."

I press a stethoscope to Mrs. DeAngelo's chest, but I hear no whoosh of air. Instead, I hear gurgling sounds, like large bubbles escaping from a pool in a hollow cavern.

Dr. Hakeem takes the stethoscope, and listens; he immediately removes the endotracheal tube. "You were in the esophagus," he says. "That was the stomach that you were hearing. An easy mistake. You must see the V-shape made by the vocal cords at the opening into the airway. If you put the tube in the esophagus, the patient will receive no oxygen; if you don't recognize and correct this, the patient will die.

"You must always check with the stethoscope after you put in an endotracheal tube," he says. "Always. Every time. No matter how sure you are that you are in the trachea."

I remember what Nathan used to say. There are few sounds in nature as beautiful as normal breath sounds.

I've seen anesthesiologists insert endotracheal tubes in patients dozens of times, but I never realized how difficult the procedure can be. I could swear that I saw the vocal cords in Mrs. DeAngelo, and that I passed the tube into the airway framed between the vocal cords—but evidently I did not. I have to line up the opening in the mouth, the vocal cords and the epiglottis, all in a straight line. It sounds so simple, but it's not so easy to do, especially if the patient is tossing and turning, and resisting insertion of the tube.

"Try intubating her again."

I try and once again I fail. And while I push the tongue aside with the laryngoscope, Hakeem cautions me about Mrs. DeAngelo's teeth.

"Be gentle. You can break a tooth with the laryngoscope and the broken fragment can go down into the lung. I've done it myself. Just once, but that was enough. The pulmonologist had to use a bronchoscope to get it out."

So many things to remember. So many ways to fail. Finally, on the fourth or fifth or hundredth attempt, I succeed in getting the tube into Mrs. DeAngelo's trachea. I listen for breath sounds with the stethoscope, and this time, I hear the glorious springtime breeze of air passing into and out of lungs. Now that we're certain we're in the airway, we remove the ambu bag, and connect the protruding end of the endotracheal tube to a large anesthesia machine. The device will breathe for Mrs. DeAngelo and deliver the inhalation anesthetic that is required.

"Practice," Dr. Hakeem says, encouraging me. "Intubate whenever you get the chance. Remember, intubate is a fabricated word. It means put a tube in, but it's the most important skill you can learn here. Later—when you're in the ICU or the Emergency Room in the middle of the night, doing CPR, or whenever a patient needs an airway—you can save their life. But you must always check the location of the tube with a stethoscope yourself. Listen to those breath sounds."

I need no convincing; my heart is still racing. What if this was the real thing, a cardiac arrest, and Mrs. DeAngelo was lying in front of us with a mouthful of saliva, clawing for oxygen while I struggled to intubate her airway and not her esophagus? Would I verify the location of the endotracheal tube in her? You bet I would. Her life would depend upon it.

Hakeem continues with what seems to be a few final words. "Even with much experience, sometimes it can be difficult. For us, as well as for you. But we're not proud. When we're in trouble, we call for help." He points to an aluminum panel on the wall behind us, within easy reach. It has an intercom speaker and two buttons. "The black button," Hakeem says, "is for routine, like to ask someone to come in when you need a bathroom break. The red one is for emergencies."

***

Dr. Peterson is just outside the operating room

where he and his team have been scrubbing their hands and forearms. They drop their scrub brushes, gown and glove and proceed with the gall bladder operation while I have the luxury of observing it all from my box seat, behind the ether screen. I'm fascinated as they begin to dissect and mobilize the gall bladder, carefully preserving the adjacent anatomic structures. And look who is here among them—Lenny Goldstein. He's third assistant, no doubt, anticipating what he will be doing when he is the surgeon.

Right now I feel an unexpected kinship with Dr. Hakeem and his fellow anesthesiologists. I never before appreciated how demanding their craft is. But as the case proceeds, I slip into a numbing routine—note the position of the airway, check the blood pressure, scan the EKG and heart rate, send an arterial blood sample for blood gases, (oxygen and carbon dioxide levels), replace an empty bag of IV fluid, and every five minutes, enter the numbers on the Anesthesia Flow Sheet— Vigilance, Vigilance. My mind drifts as the surgeons remove the gall bladder. They are having some blood loss; I'd better give some extra IV fluid. Watch the heart rate and blood pressure. Stay out of trouble.

Dr. Hakeem leaves me on my own for a few minutes. I'm alone, but I can hear his voice right outside the OR door discussing a case scheduled for tomorrow. I know he's nearby. Besides, with the anesthesia machine breathing for the patient, we're virtually on autopilot, so long as we don't disrupt the stability and location of the endotracheal tube.

Dr. Hakeem returns to the operating room. "You look sleepy," he says. "Maybe a little bored?"

I hate to admit it, but he's right. I am a little bored.

"I tell you secret of anesthesia," Hakeem says for the third or fourth time. "The real secret: Anesthesia is ninety-five percent boredom and five percent terror, and I'm not sure which is worse."

After Dr. Peterson and his residents close Mrs. DeAngelo's abdomen, we discontinue the inhalation anesthetic and wait until she can breathe on her own. Once she is able to do so, we remove the endotracheal tube, and slide her off the operating table onto a gurney. Then we wheel her into the Recovery Room where she can be closely monitored by the Recovery Room nurses.

Yes, I think to myself; ninety-five percent boredom and five percent terror.

CHAPTER 22

CRISIS IN THE OR

It's four o'clock in the afternoon and we've finished all our cases for today. But before I leave, Dr. Hakeem sends me off to see two new patients scheduled for tomorrow's surgery. Mr. Delahay and Mr. Markham are listed for the same procedures, bowel resection of a segment of the large intestine for cancer.

Mr. Delahay is a fifty-seven year old man with cancer of the large intestine, but no other known illnesses. He has no heart disease and no pulmonary problems. He looks younger than his stated age and he seems remarkably fit. He has penetrating blue eyes, small sharp features and a gray, razor-sharp crew cut. "Look," he says. "All the tests are done. We know what's in there, and that it's got to come out. Let's get on with it."

He has more resolve than most people would have in his situation. I admire him for it. I'm tempted to ask if he was in the Marines, but I think better of it.

We sit and talk for a few minutes as I rattle through my routine, explain the nature of the anesthesia he will receive, inquire about what medications he's taking and whether he has any allergies. Then I inspect his mouth for loose or false teeth, and ask him about any special needs he might have. Finally, I ask him to sign the Anesthesia Consent Document and the Blood Administration

Consent Form, in case blood transfusion becomes necessary. He scans the forms, purses his lips and puts pen to paper.

The second patient is Mr. Markham. He's a short, fifty-year old man who has, by all that's written in the chart, the same disease as Mr. Delahay. But he is a much different person. I sit at his bedside with his medical chart on my lap. He has a short, bull neck with an unusually thick, throaty voice.

"I have a really bad feeling about this," he says with a grimace.

"I'm sorry to hear that. If it makes you feel any better, I can tell you that we do this kind of surgery several times a week. It's almost routine for us."

"Routine for you," he says. "Not for me."

He's not the first patient I've encountered who has had a premonition before surgery, but I don't know what to say to reassure him. I run my finger along the edges of the pages of his chart.

"You know why you're having the surgery, I say..." But, no. I stop myself, I'm being too clinical. I try again. "If you really feel unsure, you could postpone it for a week or two..."

"Easy for you to say. I've just been through the bowel prep. Four quarts of that......well, you know. It's probably worse than the surgery. Besides, sooner or later I'm going to have to do it. Might as well do it now. ..." He brings his hands together, his fingertips touching to form a steeple.

"Has the hospital chaplain been by to see you?"

Mr. Markham shakes his head no. "Not yet."

"He will." I don't know what else to say. As I did with Mr. Delahay, I explain the details of tomorrow's anesthesia, ask Mr. Markham about allergies, and inspect his mouth for loose or false teeth. Then I ask him to sign the Anesthesia Consent Document, and the Blood Administration Consent Form. He does so slowly, reluctantly, drawing a protective ellipse around his name. I can see his jaw muscles tightening as he writes. He hands the signed document back to me. I wish him luck, shake his hand and return to the Anesthesia Department.

Dr. Hakeem is waiting for me in his office, wrapped in a gray mantle of stale cigarette smoke. "We have these two patients for tomorrow," I tell him. "Mr. Delahay and Mr. Markham." I describe the two patients and voice my concern about Mr. Markham's anxiety.

"There is not much you can say to reassure him," Dr. Hakeem says. "That's the surgeon's job. Anesthesia is very safe these days, but the patients are asleep and they have no control. For us, we do it every day; for them, it's frightening. It would be frightening for us too, if we were the patient."

I remember the discomfort I felt when Ken, Lenny and I took turns lying on the operating table, playing the role of the patient.

"There is one more thing," I tell Dr. Hakeem. "Mr. Markham is short and squat with a bull neck. I'm afraid it will be difficult to insert an endotracheal tube in his airway."

"That's an important observation," Hakeem says. "I will see them both before I leave for the evening. But first I have something for you." He takes me to the now empty pre-op holding area.

Each anesthesiologist and anesthesia resident has his own work cart, and Dr. Hakeem presents one to me as well, a bright red and aluminum Sears-Craftsman tool box on wheels. It has a wide strip of masking tape plastered across it on which he has written RESIDENT. It's filled with medications, a laryngoscope and endotracheal tubes. It's my sole possession in this place, this land of anesthesia and, even though I'm a surgical resident, for the moment I feel like a genuine member of the anesthesia team.

***

Mr. Delahay is our first case this morning. I check to be certain he received his pre-op antibiotics. He has, so we roll his gurney into the operating room, and I ask him to slide onto the operating table. After Dr. Peterson greets him, we give him the usual medications—oxygen by mask, a barbiturate and a narcotic intravenously, and an inhalation anesthetic, our standard recipe. I expect that we will use that recipe again and again.

Then I prepare to insert the endotracheal tube into his airway. I am tense as I face the challenge again, yesterday's nemesis. But unlike the difficulties I had yesterday with Mrs. DeAngelo, I can readily identify the epiglottis, the vocal cords and the entrance to the airway, and I can line them up in a straight line. The endotracheal tube slips in without difficulty. Listening to Mr. Delahay's chest, I can hear the beautiful sound of air flowing in and out of his lungs. I give Dr. Hakeem a thumbs up. I am delighted, and wonder who is more proud—Dr. Hakeem or myself. Dr Hakeem administers paralytic drugs to relax the abdominal muscles, and the surgeons begin their operation. I watch as they open the abdomen, mobilize the bowel and prepare to excise a portion of it. Lenny is there as third assistant. I'm looking forward to when I will be doing this kind of surgery.

But right now, I am serving as an anesthesiologist, not a surgical resident. Throughout the case, I monitor Mr. Delahay's progress—his EKG and pulse rate, blood pressure, and respiratory rate regulated by the anesthesia machine. I send blood for measurements of oxygen and carbon dioxide in the blood. And every five minutes I enter data on the hand-written Anesthesia Flow Sheet. The patient's well-being depends on my tracking his vital signs and responding to abnormalities promptly, before he gets into trouble. His comfort also requires that I watch for neuromuscular movements. Dr. Hakeem adds small amounts of barbiturates and narcotic as needed. This is vital as the patient, immobilized by paralytic drugs, may still feel pain and hear our conversation if he is not adequately anesthetized. It's imperative to keep him asleep and free of pain. It's a serious responsibility, but it's repetitive and gradually it becomes monotonous.

After an hour and a half, the portion of the bowel

harboring the tumor is removed, and the surgeons have sewn the free ends of the transected bowel back together to re-establish continuity. Now the surgeons begin to close the abdomen. They talk among themselves about the procedure and the fact that the liver looked clean without evidence of metastases. At the same time, Dr. Hakeem guides me as we reduce the anesthetic medications. Mr. Delahay begins to awaken. When he is able to breathe on his own, we remove the endotracheal tube and talk with him to be certain he's awake. When we are sure, we slide him onto a gurney brought next to the operating table. Then we wheel him into the Recovery Room. In every way, this has been a satisfying procedure, and I do hope the surgery was performed in time, before the tumor has spread.

***

While the custodians clean and mop the room for the next case, I visit with Mr. Markham in the pre-op holding area. The routine pre-op Valium we give to all the patients has mollified much of his anxiety, and he seems to have much less foreboding than he did last night. I shake his hand, and assure him that things will be fine, but candidly, I'm not so sure. I'm still worried about his short bull neck. How am I going to get the endotracheal tube through there?

I check to be certain that he received his pre-op antibiotics. He has. Accordingly, we roll Mr. Markham on his gurney into the operating room, and I ask him to slide over onto the operating table. Dr. Peterson greets him. Then Peterson leaves the room to take a phone call as we begin to administer our regular concoction of anesthetic agents—oxygen by mask, a barbiturate and a narcotic intravenously, and an inhalation anesthetic.

When he is asleep, Dr. Hakeem and I open his mouth, and I search for the vocal cords that will lead me to his airway. But his jaw is stiff and resistant to manipulation, and his short neck makes it difficult to see straight through to the back of his throat. Dr. Hakeem gives Mr. Markham a paralytic agent to relax his neck

175

and jaw muscles, and permit us to open his mouth widely. But the medication also suppresses his respiration. When I stare into the back of his throat, I cannot visualize his cords or the entrance to his airway. I search for five or ten seconds. No luck. My hands are trembling with anxiety. All the while, Mr. Markham is not breathing. How long can he go without taking a breath? My heart is racing.

"Here," Hakeem says, taking the laryngoscope. "Let me have a look."

He searches quickly, but is also is unsuccessful. Even worse, my manipulation of the soft tissues in the back of his throat with the laryngoscope has caused them to bleed slightly and to swell, further obscuring our view. Dr. Hakeem hurriedly connects the football-shaped Ambu Bag onto a mask that covers Mr. Markham's nose and mouth. Hakeem rhythmically squeezes the bag to ventilate the patient, but he can move only a small amount of air into and out of the lungs. We must act quickly as Mr. Markham's skin is turning blue, and his heart rate is up to 120 beats per minute. Dr. Hakeem tries repeatedly to intubate him, but he is unsuccessful. Poor Mr. Markham—he has come to the operating room; he has brought his premonitions with him, and they seem to be coming true.

The EKG shows that his pulse is now almost 150 beats per minute with some ominous-looking abnormal electrical activity. His skin is an alarming shade of blue, and we still cannot oxygenate him effectively, even with the hand-held Ambu bag. Dr. Hakeem reaches back to the aluminum intercom panel on the wall and presses the red button, the emergency call for help. Within seconds, Dr. Chung bursts into the room along with Dr. Mukergee, another attending anesthesiologist.

"I can't intubate him," Hakeem cries. "And I'm having trouble ventilating him."

Dr. Chung stands transfixed for a moment, taking in the scene before him. Then he grabs the laryngoscope from Hakeem, and takes a position at the head of the operating table. He hyperextends Mr. Markham's neck as far back as it will go. His gaze is locked on the anatomy in the back of Mr. Markham's throat. I don't know just what he can see back there, but without taking his eye from it, he reaches out with his free right hand and motions frantically for the endotracheal tube. Dr. Hakeem passes it to him, and Chung hurriedly inserts it into what hopefully is the airway. The endotracheal tube is in, but in where?

Hakeem connects an Ambu Bag to the end of the endotracheal tube, and rhythmically squeezes oxygen into it. I listen to Mr. Markham's chest with a stethoscope, and I am pleased...no, thrilled, to hear the sound of air whooshing to and fro, in and out of his lungs. There is not a hint of the bubbling sound that I heard when I put the tube in Mrs. DeAngelo's esophagus. I stand back and watch Mr. Markham's pulse gradually fall to less than a hundred beats per minute, and his color change from a distressed blue to pink.

My heart is still racing. "How did you do it?" I ask Dr. Chung.

He turns toward me, and answers with a kaleidoscope of Chinese-American babble. I haven't the slightest idea of what he is saying, but whatever it is, I am grateful that he is as skilled as he is, and that he is here. I have nothing but respect for that man.

As the tension in the room subsides, the door swings open and an irate Dr. Peterson comes prancing in on his high horse. "You guys done fooling around?"

"You can start any time you want to," Hakeem says, putting on a calm face before the surgeon.

"It's about time," Peterson says in spite of the fact that it was he who spent all this time on the telephone while we struggled to intubate his patient.

"By the way," Hakeem adds. "He was a very difficult intubation, Very difficult." His Arabic accent and the recent turn of events strongly flavor his words. "I don't think we could intubate him again. Next time, you may have to do a tracheotomy. Your residents must not dislodge the tube whether or not we are present. We must decide when it is time to remove the tube."

Dr. Peterson nods. In spite of all his irate bravura, he gets the message.

From that point on, Mr. Markham's surgery goes smoothly, and there is no obvious evidence of spread of the tumor. At the end of the case, we stop giving the anesthetic agents, but leave the endotracheal tube in place for overnight. We want to wait until we are convinced that he is fully awake, and the full complement of Anesthesia and Surgical Staff is present and available. I am relieved to see him awaken with no apparent neurological deficits. And thank goodness for Dr. Chung, difficult to understand, but truly a wizard.

Ninety-five percent boredom and five percent terror. Hakeem wasn't exaggerating when he said that. I had my ninety-five percent boredom earlier, and now I've had my five percent terror. I wonder how many more of these crises I'm going to have to endure over the course of my three-month rotation on Anesthesia. And what if I was an anesthesiologist and I was alone, without Dr. Hakeem or Dr. Chung? Then what? These are brave fellows, these anesthesiologists.

I finish up my work and make a pre-op visit to a patient who is scheduled for a hernia repair tomorrow. How grateful I am to have a routine case. I get the patient's signature on the Anesthesia Consent Form. Before I leave the hospital, I stop in to see Mr. Markham. He is sitting up in bed, awake and alert, complaining of post-op pain. His family is in his room with him, and he seems to be in good spirits for a man who just had major surgery and a difficult intubation, and he doesn't know the half of it.

CHAPTER 23

FIRST NIGHT IN THE ER

I am sitting in the medical records department dictating a discharge summary when my pager goes off directing me to call Dr. Loring, the Chief of the Emergency Room.

"I'm calling you about working in the ER," he says. "We're always looking for people to work in the ER, and we thought you might like to consider it."

"Well, I'm not sure. I'll be a senior (fifth year resident) in a couple of months, and I expect to be very busy. What will I do if I'm faced with a crucial decision, and I *zig* when I should have *zagged*?"

"As a senior, you will be busy," Loring concedes. "But you'll probably do some moonlighting here or at some other hospital. Everybody does and this is just about the easiest ER you'll ever work in. If you work at another hospital, you'll be responsible for everyone who walks in the door— pediatrics, cardiology—everything."

He's right about that.

"Here, we're a university hospital, so you have all kinds of support. If a patient comes in with a cardiac problem, you can call the second-year internal medicine resident and he'll admit and manage him. If he's over his head, he can ask the cardiology fellow to come in from home. And that's true for ENT (ear, nose, and throat), Ophthalmology, and all the medical disciplines. So you would have lots of backup."

PHILIP B. DOBRIN, M.D.

I mull over what Loring says, and it makes sense. Still...I'm not sure.

"The salary," Loring adds, "is twenty-five dollars an hour, plus we pay the malpractice premiums."

"Twenty-five dollars an hour! Sounds better every minute—when do I start?"

"We will schedule you for twice a month—an eight hour shift every other weekend, when you wouldn't have any regularly scheduled surgery. Your first stint would be from eleven on Saturday night to seven Sunday morning. How's that sound?"

"It all sounds good, and twenty-five dollars an hour sounds *wonderful.*"

***

On Saturday night, I arrive at the ER just before eleven to meet Nikki and Alyssa, the two regular night nurses. Nikki is a pleasant, dark-haired woman in her mid-forties with many years of experience. Alyssa is a few years older, with coarse pock-marked skin, a raspy voice and a crusty personality to match. They're tough ol' birds who have worked in the ER since University Hospital opened. I've heard from other residents that both are extremely competent. I'm sure I'll learn a lot from them.

Alyssa takes me around to see the examining rooms. There are five in all, and they are all about the same—abbreviated operating rooms where one can examine patients and perform minor surgical procedures.

"Just look at how small these rooms are." Alyssa says disapprovingly.

I don't know what she's crabbing about. The examining rooms look fine to me. Of course, this is her domain, and I guess her opinion depends on what her expectations are.

We finish our tour at a small room at the end of the corridor. "This is your call room when you work down here. Some nights you may be lucky and get a few hours sleep."

It's a tiny room, just large enough for a three foot wide bed and a diminutive desk. There's also a view box on the wall for examining x-ray films. Actually, I don't

180

expect to be doing much sleeping when I'm working down here.

We return to the nurses' station. "There are no patients now," Alyssa says. "But it's Saturday night, and your welcoming committee will be here soon enough."

She introduces me to Yolanda, a dark-haired Hispanic receptionist who greets the patients when they arrive. Her job is to smile and obtain the patient's insurance information. Her bilingual skills and pleasant personality must be invaluable.

Finally, Alyssa takes me to the break room. It's really a cramped linen closet with folded sheets, blankets and towels piled higher and higher on shelves all the way up to the drop ceiling. There's also a tiny table with three chairs.

"It's like a john in an airplane," Alyssa says. "So small there isn't room to change your mind." She gives me a blast of her cackling, ex-smokers laugh.

"This is our coffee break room." Nikki points to a percolating aluminum pot that's bathing the cramped space with the aroma of fresh coffee.

"Help yourself," Alyssa says. "The empty coffee can on the top shelf is the kitty. Feed the kitty—if you can reach it."

There's that cackling laugh again. I reach into my pocket to feel for some money to contribute, but my wallet is in my locker in the OR.

"Sometimes we send out for pizza," Alyssa says. "You're welcome to join us for that, too." Then she turns abruptly, and walks away.

Nikki remains, assessing me with a vacant look.

"Don't mind Alyssa," she says. "She pissed at having to train new residents all the time. Just about the time we teach them how we do things around here, they leave and we have to start over again. It's nothing personal."

At eleven-fifteen, we receive our first patient, Elliott Marks. Nikki puts him in Examining Room One. According to the ER admission sheet, he was playing softball at the company picnic Saturday afternoon, and twisted his ankle.

"It happened hours ago," his wife says. She's a frazzled black-haired scarecrow of a woman who is proud that she convinced her husband to come to the ER.

"It was the company picnic, so we'll be covered by their insurance. "Right, Doc? Right?" She looks expectantly at me.

"I'm not sure," I tell her. "Billing is not my specialty. I kneel down to feel Mr. Marks's swollen ankle. "How did you do this?"

"Trying to stretch a single into a double."

"Were you safe or out?"

"Safe."

"Then it probably was worth it."

"I'm not so sure. They beat us anyway, twenty-one to fourteen."

"Twenty-one to fourteen! Sounds like a pitchers' duel with me pitching for both sides."

Mr. Marks begins to laugh.

Finally. I get a smile out of somebody.

I look down at Mr. Marks's swollen ankle, but without an x-ray, I can't be sure whether or not there's a fracture. "We need an x-ray," I tell him.

Nikki puts Mr. Marks in a wheelchair and takes him down to the X-ray department. Twenty minutes later, he's back with a film on his lap. Attached is a reading provided by the Radiology resident. He is here until midnight. His report reads *Soft tissue injury with edema (swelling). No evidence of fracture.*

I put the film up on the view box in the examining room, and squint at what might be fracture lines. When I'm convinced there are none, I wrap the ankle with an Ace bandage, apply an ice bag, and give him some crutches. I offer to write a prescription for pain medication, but he says he doesn't need it.

"I want you to elevate your leg," I tell him. "And return to Orthopedics clinic next week. It's going to take about six weeks to heal. Try to stay off it, and keep it higher than your heart. Fluid flows downhill. If you keep it elevated, you will minimize the swelling."

"I'll put it up on a pillow," he says.

"No, that's not good enough. You'll mash down the pillow, and kick it off the bed in your sleep. Better to put phone books under the foot of the bed. It will give you reliable elevation."

"I'll do it," he says. "But six weeks to heal. Isn't there something I can do to speed that up?"

"Sorry. The only treatment I know of for an over-stretched ligament is *Tincture of time.*"

"Tincture of time," Mr. Marks says. Rolling the words on the tip of his tongue. "I like the sound of that." He thanks me for my attention, and leaves the ER with the scarecrow at his side carrying on about how smart he was for listening to her and visiting the Emergency Room, and how he has to keep his leg elevated and not just use a pillow and how it's not broken but the ligaments are stretched. And the door closes behind them.

Phew. Silence prevails.

After she has gone, I lean against the counter to catch my breath, (if there's any unused oxygen left.)

Then I ask Nikki, "Who reads the films after midnight, when the Radiology resident has gone home?"

"You do, but a Radiology attending goes over all the night films first thing in the morning. Whenever we miss something, we call the patients at home, and have them come back. And it does happen occasionally."

She makes it sound like an everyday occurrence. That gives me some comfort, but not much.

"And we call *all* the ER patients on the second or third day," she says. "Just to see how they're doing."

***

At one o'clock, a Mr. Mardel comes in with chest pain radiating down his left arm and up the left side of his jaw. He's pale, sweaty and short of breath. These are all signs consistent with an acute myocardial infarction, an MI, a heart attack. We rush him into Examining Room One, bypassing Yolanda and her onerous insur-

183

ance forms. We connect Mr. Mardel to the EKG machine and deliver oxygen with a small plastic tube inserted in his nostrils. We also start an IV in a vein in his arm. I check the consultation listings, and see that Alan Brofsky is on tonight. He's a good-natured resident designated to provide Internal Medicine skills in the ER, when they are needed.

"Better call Brofsky," I say to Alyssa.

"Done," she answers curtly.

Alan Brofsky is finishing his second year on internal medicine, and from watching him assess Mr. Mardel, it is evident that he has spent considerable time on Cardiology. After he examines Mr. Mardel, he steps out of the examining room to call the cardiology fellow at home. I listen in to their conversation as they discuss the patient's condition. The fellow agrees to come in to see Mr. Mardel, and Brofsky will transfer him to the Coronary ICU.

Dr. Loring was right. This isn't that bad. Not only that, Mr. Mardel is being cared for by expert internists and cardiologists, not by a moonlighting surgical resident posing as an internist. It's one of the advantages to patients coming to a university teaching hospital. If I were acutely ill, that's where I would choose to go.

****

At one a.m., a young mother with a feverish squalling infant comes into the Emergency Room. Alyssa calls Dr. Patel, the Pediatrics resident on call. She assesses the baby and, after speaking with her attending by phone, decides to do a spinal tap to rule out meningitis. Then she admits the child to Pediatrics. There is nothing for me to do but the paperwork.

***

At two a.m., Mr. Hayes brings his seventy-five year old father to the Emergency Room for shortness of breath. The father lives alone, and his son found him on the floor confused and disoriented. We immediately give him supplementary oxygen by nasal cannulas, and I prepare to start an IV line. At the same time, Nikki pages

Dr. Brofsky. The son stands by, watching as I am about to insert a needle into a vein in his father's arm. Without warning, the older man pulls a pistol out of his jacket pocket and begins waving it wildly over our heads. "I hate those needles," he says. "So you'd better not hurt me."

"Give me the gun, pop," the son says. But the father keeps the weapon, waving it over his head, just out of his son's reach. Everyone ducks out of the examining room while father and son tussle over the weapon. Finally, the son wrests the gun away from his father, and everyone returns to the patient.

"Sonny," the old man grumbles. "You've got the gun, now. You watch them real close. If they hurt me, *you* shoot them."

At that moment, the hospital guards and Alan Brofsky arrive. In just a few seconds we learn that the handgun is not loaded, and that Brofsky knows Mr. Hayes from Internal Medicine outpatient clinic. Brofsky makes a few phone calls and he admits the confused old man to the ICU. Nikki gives the handgun to the policemen.

When the excitement calms down, I ask Alyssa, "Have you ever seen that before, I mean with a gun and all?"

"Sure," Alyssa says. "Happens all the time."

"You're kidding...Right? All the time!"

Alyssa walks away.

***

At three-thirty, Mr. and Mrs. Thomas, a mature black couple, arrives at the Emergency Room. They are stylishly dressed to see the doctor, even at this late hour. Mr. Thomas wears a freshly ironed white shirt and suit jacket, while Mrs. Thomas wears a black dress with a decorative gold pin. That's a degree of formality that we rarely see at University ER or clinic. They are here because Mr. Thomas claims that he feels a foreign body in the back of his throat.

"I made fish for dinner," Mrs. Thomas says. "Perch, Arthur's favorite. But now he says he can feel a bone stuck in his throat. He says he can't see anything when he looks in the mirror. I've looked, but I can't see anything either. Still he insists there's something there."

I lead Mr. and Mrs. Thomas into Examining Room Three where I use a bright lamp to examine Mr. Thomas's throat. But even using a tongue depressor to push the tongue and soft tissues aside, I cannot see very far back in the throat. I certainly cannot visualize any foreign object. Mr. Thomas coughs and repeatedly tries to clear his throat.

Finally, I leave the examining room to call Bill Timmins, the Ear, Nose and Throat resident on call. I relay Mr. Thomas's complaints, and describe my attempts to identify a foreign object. "This guy needs indirect laryngoscopy," I tell Timmins "That's the only way we'll be able to see far enough back in there."

But Bill is not eager to come in at three o'clock in the morning to search for what may prove to be a phantom fishbone. "There's probably nothing there," he says. "Probably just some irritation that feels like something. We see it all the time."

"Maybe so," I say. "But these people got up in the middle of the night, got dressed in their Sunday best and came into the ER. They are going to be charged for an ER visit, and I think they're entitled to the best treatment we have to offer. Unfortunately, that's not me. It's ENT."

Timmins hems and haws, hoping I'll back down. But I don't.

I have to admit I'm frustrated. Some of the subspecialty residents like ENT get called so infrequently that they almost never have to come into the hospital. That's a privilege not shared by those of us in General Surgery and Internal Medicine. So be it. But when the guys in ENT *do* get called, I feel they should come in without making a fuss about it. What Timmins doesn't realize is that if he refuses to come in, I have every intention of calling his attending at home. I can imagine the mood of the attending over being awakened at three o'clock in the morning to search for an evanescent fishbone after a resident refused to come in. I suspect he would have a few words with me as well as Timmins. It won't make me very popular with the ENT residents, but it's their responsibility.

At last, Timmins agrees to come in. When he arrives, he immediately begins grousing about needing to examine Mr. Thomas in the ENT clinic where he has all his instruments and good lighting. Alyssa pages one of the night guards and asks him to unlock the door to the Ear, Nose and Throat Clinic. I accompany them when they walk over. There, Timmins expertly inserts some probes with mirrors into Mr. Thomas's throat; they permit him to see deep into the recesses of the throat. In just a few seconds he identifies a translucent fishbone, the length and thickness of a straight pin caught in the soft tissue on the right side of his throat. Taking care not to drop it back in the throat, he cautiously removes it. He is beaming when he shows the culprit to Mr. and Mrs. Thomas who seem delighted to see it.

"See," Mr. Thomas says to his wife. "I told you there was something in there."

Timmins schedules Mr. Thomas for a return visit to ENT clinic in two days, and sends him on his way. I want to thank Timmins for coming in, but I can't find him. Alyssa tells me he's already gone home to bed.

Then it occurs to me—I should have tried to use a laryngoscope to push the tongue aside and visualize the lower regions of the throat, like when intubating the airway. Of course, grabbing and extracting that flimsy bone might not have been so easy. And dropping it back down into the throat or, worse yet, dropping it back into the airway could have turned it into a serious problem. But wait, I've got to stop second-guessing myself. I'm glad I called Timmins, and he got the job done without complications.

CHAPTER 24

FULL MOON OVER THE EMERGENCY ROOM

It's 10:45 in the evening and I take a short cut through the parking lot to the Emergency Room. My path is lit by a full and luminous moon. When I get to the ER, Nikki and Alyssa are already there.

"Did you see that moon?" Alyssa asks. "A full moon like that is going to fire up every psych patient in the county."

"You don't believe those old wives' tales, do you?"

"You'll see," she says with a sly smile. "If we can see that moon, they can too."

The ER has just one patient, Mr. Lewis, in Examining Room One. Alyssa tells me that Mr. Lewis was struck by an automobile while riding his bicycle on a dark, tree-lined street. "He has a fracture of his fibula, the smaller bone in his left lower leg. It was set and casted by Tom French, the Orthopedics resident." According to Alyssa, Mr. Lewis's behavior has been very strange.

I enter Examining Room One to see for myself, where I am greeted by a garrulous monologue of rhythmic words and phrases.

"The moon grows wider every day, they slip and slick and mooney rick...."

There, I find a disheveled-looking, middle-aged man sitting upright on a gurney with a cast on his left leg. His hair is wild and uncombed, and he is chattering breathlessly, pouring out a stream of disconnected rhymes and phrases. The floor is covered with sheets of a ring-bound notebook that lies in his lap. Each page has a few illegible words scrawled on it before it sails off to the floor. This guy really is not just strange; he's floridly manic.

Mr. Lewis glances up without acknowledging my presence or interrupting his monologue.

"Oil rigs are rumpled red. They're parked nearby as well they should..."

"Tell me, Mr. Lewis, do you have family at home?"

He shakes his head *no* and keeps on talking.

"Where do you live, Mr. Lewis?"

"On Second Street. Behind the gas station." He waves his hand above his head, and gulps a mouthful of air.

It's the first time I've seen him take a breath "In an apartment?" I ask.

"No, in a Chevy."

"In a Chevy? Why do you live in a Chevy?"

"Cause it's got a better heater than a Buick."

I'll take his word for it.

"Do you have family?" I ask again.

He says *no*, but nods *yes,* and he keeps on talking.

That's enough for me. "Just sit tight, Mr. Lewis." I give him a reassuring pat. "We'll have Dr. Rabin see you. He's the psychiatry resident on call tonight. I know you're going to like him. As a matter of fact, in some ways you two speak the same language."

Mr. Lewis nods, and returns to the Declaration of Independence, or whatever it was he was reciting.

I leave Mr. Lewis and return to the nurses' station. "Better call the psych resident," I say to Alyssa." This guy, Lewis. He's really manic."

Alyssa gets on the phone to page Dr. Rabin. "Doctor," she says loud enough for me to hear her. "We need you in the ER. We have a *full moon special.*"

It takes twenty minutes before Dr. Rabin honors us with his presence. He's a portly, balding fellow who was in practice in Family Medicine before he discovered that his patients required psychiatric care more than they needed his medical attention. That's when he decided to do two extra years of residency in Psychiatry.

Dr. Rabin is in his early forties. He strolls his way into the Emergency Room without exhibiting the slightest rush. He walks with a slightly comical, leaning back posture with toes pointed upward and outward. He plops his bulky abdomen against the counter top in the nurses' station and listens to my description of Mr. Lewis, and our discussion of the relative merits of Chevys versus Buicks.

Dr. Rabin listens intently. "He's not in restraints, is he?"

"Oh, no, he's not dangerous to himself or others, he's just manic."

The overuse of restraints has become an issue of nationwide concern in Psychiatric circles, and it is one of Rabin's pet peeves. "Good," he says, as he disappears into Examining Room One.

While Rabin is examining Mr. Lewis, an ambulance arrives at our door to deliver a violent psychiatric patient strapped to an ambulance gurney. His family arrives separately in their own car. From the family we learn that the patient, Jerrold Williams, has been using a concoction of recreational drugs, including large amounts of cocaine. These street drugs are known to cause serious abnormal heart rhythms. We put Mr. Williams in Examining Room Two, connect him to an EKG monitor, and restrain him with leather straps. Nikki and Alyssa check him every ten or fifteen minutes to be sure that the restraints are not too tight.

Unbeknownst to us, Dr. Rabin hears the hub-bub in the hall. He briefly leaves Mr. Lewis and slips into Examining Room Two. There, he examines Mr. Williams, and finds him sleeping quietly. Rabin decides that the now calm patient is ready to be released from restraints. He removes them, and then goes off to the break room to get a cup of coffee. He is just returning when a newly energized Mr. Williams, drug-crazed and apparently hallucinating, tears out of Examining Room Two, races down the hall nearly naked to crash head-on into Dr. Rabin in the corridor. The usually impassive psychiatrist is suddenly entangled with churning legs and scalding coffee as everyone in the Emergency Room dashes down the corridor to give assistance.

Alyssa is furious with Dr. Rabin for releasing Mr. Williams without discussing doing so with the ER staff.

"That guy is crazy," Rabin shouts. "Cray—Zee."

"Is that your official diagnosis, Dr. Rabin?" Alyssa asks.

"You bet it is," he says, doing his best to wipe hot coffee off his neck and collar. "Cray—Zee."

We get Mr. Williams into a hospital gown, back on a gurney and into leather restraints, and Dr. Rabin agrees to see both Mr. Lewis and Mr. Williams.

***

At one a.m., Tom French, the orthopedic resident, stops by to check on Mr. Lewis. Tom is a strapping ex-athlete who played college football before he went to medical school.

He and Rabin are about as different as two men could be, one being highly conceptual, the other practical and concrete. It is purely by chance that they both are on in-hospital call the same night, but they provide an entertaining contrast.

"Do you orthopods fine-tune your surgical skills on the weekends by chopping wood?" Rabin asks.

"As a matter of fact, we do," Tom says. "But we don't treat invisible diseases that nobody can see on x-ray like you guys do."

Tom walks into Examining Room One to check on Mr. Lewis, but he's out in a flash, holding his nose. "Do you know what that goof ball did? He pissed into his cast. It stinks in there."

"What are you going to do?" I ask Tom. "Make a new cast?"

"Oh no, not tonight, I'm not. Maybe tomorrow, after we finish our cases. Maybe never. In the meantime, he can stew in his own juices."

"*Stew in his own juices.* Please," Nikki says. "Must you put it that way?"

"I guess you'll just have to watch him," Rabin says.

"I'm not watching him," Tom says indignantly. "And I'm not taking him on our service. He has a fracture. We treated that. Now his problem is that he's a nut case. He's yours, Rabin. I'll stop by and see him every day, but I'm not doing his History and Physical, and I'm sure as hell not going to do his Discharge Summary."

Everybody hates the paper work.

I watch as Rabin starts to object, but then he acquiesces. Tom is right, and Rabin knows it. Mr. Lewis has a fractured fibula, but his real problem lies above his shoulders.

***

It's two a.m., and right now the ER is quiet. However, there's a State Mental Health facility nearby, and their staff routinely sends us their patients who have medical problems. When patients are sent to the ER, they are always accompanied by a glib orderly named Louie. He's short and energetic with spiky black hair that points outward in all directions, like the Statue of Liberty.

At two-thirty, Louie brings us a forty-five year old patient named Albert Burns. Apparently the ER staff is well-acquainted with Mr. Burns's psychiatric history, and everyone working in the ER repeats Mr. Burns's Scottish name while heavily rolling their r's. When I first meet him, Mr. Burns is sitting on the edge of a gurney, filled with antipsychotic medications, and glowing the soft smile of a man who is truly at peace. Louie stands beside him.

"Do you know this patient?" I ask Louie.

"Of course, I know this patient. It is part of my cushy state job to know our patients." He stops mid-munch on a walnut-size mouthful of pink bubble gum. Then he continues. "Burns's roommate, Mr. Houghton, says he's been missing a quarter for the last three days. He thinks Burnsie here ate it." Louie pops a huge pink bubble, and starts laughing.

"What's so funny," I ask.

"I don't know. It's just funny. Eating his roommate's quarter."

I turn to the patient. "Is that true, Mr. Burns? Did you eat your roommate's quarter?"

Mr. Burns stares off into space. Not much to be learned here.

Back to Louie. "You know, even if he did swallow a quarter a few days ago, it'll probably get through all right. Especially if we give him some mineral oil to grease the skids."

Louie works on his gum.

"Of course," I say, "we're not even sure there's anything in there. Why don't we get an x-ray and find out." I write the order, and send Mr. Burns and Louie off to the X-ray Department.

After about twenty minutes, Louie returns to the Emergency Room with a broad grin and Mr. Burns in tow. Louie carries a large X-ray film under his arm. It's a view of Mr. Burns's abdomen.

I put the film up on the illuminated view box in the ER, and we study it carefully. I see no quarters, but I do spot three smaller, round metal discs in the abdomen, somewhere in the small intestine.

Louie sidles up beside me. "Mind if I have a look?"

"Not at all. What do you think you see there, Louie?"

"No quarter, but *there*." He points to the three metal discs on the X-ray film. "It looks like two dimes and a nickel."

"Looks that way."

"Hey. This guy's a living change machine!"

"I think you're right. So now, Louie, your work is cut out for you. You're going to have to watch this guy to make sure he doesn't swallow anything else."

"I can do that."

"And you must be sure that everything that went in comes out—you're going to have to inspect his bowel movements."

Louie looks at me with wide eyes, pretending to gag on his gum.

"Not only that, with those three coins in there, you're going to have to strain his stool to make sure you can find all of them."

" Louie shakes his head. No way."

"But it's part of your cushy state job. Those coins could obstruct his bowel. They could perforate his bowel. They could kill him."

Louie shrugs. "If he dies, he dies—I'm not touching his shit. Not even with rubber gloves. That's not part of my job. Besides, I didn't tell him to swallow the stupid quarters."

"Nickels and dimes."

"Nickels and dimes."

"Well, I'm going to have to write my recommendations in my report for your supervisor, the sheet you take back with you." I carefully write out my report, and hand it to Louie. Under "Recommendations" I write:

1. 30 cc of mineral oil by mouth each day for three days.

2. Examine stool with each bowel movement.

3. Check patient for symptoms of obstruction each shift.

4. Return to ER in two days for follow-up.

Louie sits next to Mr. Burns, and works fiercely on his gum. He blows a colossal transparent bubble. It pops. Louie peels it off his face, and then continues chewing the shattered bubble.

I let him ruminate for a few minutes while I review the lab data for Mr. Lewis and Jerrold Williams. Finally, I say as solemnly as I can, "Of course, Louis, if Mr. Burns has no symptoms for the next couple of days, we probably could forget about inspecting the stool, and just get another x-ray to see if the three coins are still there."

Louis glares at me, his face turning florid red. "You knew you were going to do that all along. I just know you did." He pulls Mr. Burns by the arm, and drags him back to the Mental Health facility van.

"Why did you eat those coins, Burnsie?" Louis asks, his face just inches away from Mr. Burns's face. "You see what trouble you got us into?"

"And don't forget the mineral oil," I call to him. "It's in my recommendations."

***

At four a.m., an ambulance drives up the Emergency Room ramp to deliver Mr. Link, a patient whose medical and psychiatric history are well-known to the doctors at University Hospital. Mr. Link is shocking even to our jaded Emergency Room Staff when they realize that he deliberately cut his hand off at the wrist. He did so at home on a band saw, and the ambulance crew brings the severed hand wrapped in ice with them. We type and cross-match Mr. Link for possible blood transfusion, get his labs and call Paul Linwood, the Hand Surgery fellow on call. Linwood is a lanky fellow with an agreeable manner, even at this late hour. He arrives in the ER, and goes immediately into Examining Room Three, and then he pops out almost as quickly as he went in.

"He refuses to sign the consent form for us to re-implant the hand," he says. "And he says if we do it against his will, he'll sue us and cut it off again. This guy is really a nut case."

Rabin quickly interviews the patient while Linwood consults by phone with his attending at home. A few minutes later, Linwood and Rabin return to the nurses' station.

The group of us gathers to make some decisions.

"He's not out of touch with reality," Rabin says. "He didn't hear voices telling him to cut his hand off or anything like that, but he's very angry and he's punishing himself. It's a form of self-mutilation. He may not be hearing voices, but cutting your hand off on a band saw is not normal behavior either, no matter how angry you are."

"So-o-o," Linwood asks. "What is it? Is he crazy or not?"

"Sort of yes, and sort of no."

"Geeze," Linwood says, throwing his hands up and over his head. "Sounds like something a psychiatrist would say."

"So what are you going to do?" I ask Linwood.

"My attending is not going to operate on anybody who refuses to sign a consent."

We all think for a moment.

Linwood nods his head. "We can't just operate on someone against their will who *may* be psychotic. That would be assault and battery."

"How about if we call a judge?" I ask.

"No good," Alyssa says. "We've done that in the past, and it takes hours to hear back from them."

"But if we wait for the patient to change his mind, the hand will be useless," Linwood says.

"I'm going to call the Chief of Staff," I say. "He's the top Doc in the hospital. Maybe he'll give us administrative permission to operate. I hate to see this guy lose his hand."

We awaken the Chief of Staff who listens to our dilemma. He doesn't dither for a moment as he agrees to give us administrative permission to re-implant the hand. "Let him sue me," he says. "What judge in this country is going to censure me for trying save some loony's perfectly good hand?"

"Hey, Linwood," I say. "I just spoke with the Chief of Staff. He said we can go ahead."

"He did? What if the patient sues us?"

"The Chief of Staff says that no judge is going to come after us for saving a patient's perfectly good hand."

"That's easy for him to say. He's not the one doing the surgery and the one likely to get sued. Is he a lawyer?"

"Not that I know of."

This is all getting very complicated. Linwood gets on the phone to speak with his reluctant attending. After discussing it between themselves, they agree that neither of them is willing to operate without a *bona fide* signed consent. The Hand Surgery attending agrees to come in and be here if the patient changes his mind, but they will operate only if they have the patient's approval in writing, no matter what the Chief of Staff says. Linwood and Nikki decide to wheel Mr. Link to the operating room where the anesthesiologists will see him. They can prepare him for surgery there, just in case he does change his mind.

A moment after they leave, Alyssa goes chasing after them. "Hey, Linwood." she shouts. "Wait up. You forgot his hand!"

The ER is suddenly quiet, and I'm feeling uncertain about what we're doing. Maybe I'd better call a judge after all or at least show that I *tried* to reach one.

CHAPTER 25

THE PLASTIC SURGEON IN THE ER

The Emergency Room is quiet until two o'clock in the morning when Miss Marilyn O'Connor drives up to the ER entrance ramp. She is an elegant lady in her early forties with a rich Carolina drawl and a fluttering southern charm. She's here because she has an uneven two centimeter-long gash on her right forearm, cut on a broken glass while she was washing dishes.

"At two o'clock in the morning?" I ask.

"I like things tidy," she says. "I couldn't bear the thought of going to bed, and leaving dirty dishes in the sink all night." Miss O'Connor has sculpted red hair and, in spite of the late hour, she is wearing bright red lipstick.

Nikki cleanses and soaks the injured arm in a solution of iodine in saline, a solution that should sterilize the wound. She makes certain that Miss O'Connor's tetanus immunization is up-to-date. Then she opens a minor surgical tray to provide the instruments I'll need to close the wound. Before beginning, I give Miss O'Connor a consent form to read and sign.

She looks up with a concerned frown. "How many stitches will it need?"

"Oh, three. Maybe four."

"Will it hurt?"

"A little, but not much. We'll make it numb, like at the dentist."

She nods. "Will it leave a scar?"

"Yes, but it should be small."

"I don't want a big scar." She absently pats her perfect red hair. "Doctor, do you think it will become infected?"

"Miss O'Conner. The injury occurred in a sink full of clean, soapy water. You couldn't ask for a better place to cut yourself. It's very unlikely to become infected. I think it will heal just fine, possibly with just a small scar."

"Can you be sure?"

"Well, there are no guarantees in medicine. But if you haven't had wound-healing problems in the past, I wouldn't expect any problems now."

Nevertheless, we've all heard horror stories of litigious patients who claimed not to be informed, and seem never to be happy, no matter what we do, and what the outcome of treatment. I bring Nikki into the room to act as a witness, and I explain everything in detail again to Miss O'Connor.

She cocks her head, and listens intently. When I finish, she stares at me and asks, "Are you a plastic surgeon?"

"No ma'am. I'm a fourth year resident in General Surgery."

"Oh, just General Surgery."

"Not *just* General Surgery," I say suppressing a wave of irritation. "Four years of abdominal surgery—hernias, gall bladders, intestines—real operations."

She shrugs. "When you operate on somebody, do you leave a scar?"

"Yes ma'am, every time. Whenever someone cuts their skin, it *always* leaves a scar. That's the way we heal."

No matter how complex the surgery is internally, the only part the patient sees is the skin incision and, later, the scar. Even if we save a patient's life with surgical heroics, often it's the appearance of the scar that counts the most to them. How often have I heard a patient say—"Dr. Smith, he's a fine doctor. Look what a small scar he made."

By now, I'm not at all interested in closing this vain lady's wound, but it's nearly three o'clock in the morning, and I am the doctor responsible for the Emergency Room.

"I want a Plastic Surgeon," she says.

"Unfortunately, there are no plastic surgeons in the house at this hour."

"Can't you call one in?"

"I can, but they usually come in only for emergencies."

"Emergencies? Like what?"

"Like life-threatening body burns, like re-attaching severed fingers…"

"But *this* is an emergency." She looks down at the modest cut on her arm, and then extends her arm toward me. "I don't want a scar."

Not what I'd call life-threatening, but I understand. She's entitled to ask for whatever she wants. Whether or not I can provide it—well, that might be another story.

"I'll try to reach someone," I say as I go to the phone.

The attending plastic surgeon on call tonight is Dr. Wisniewski, the chief of plastic surgery. I ask him if he is interested in coming to see this patient.

"Are you nuts?" he bellows. "It's three o'clock in the morning. I'm not going to get up and come into the emergency room to put in three lousy stitches in some vain woman's arm. Close it yourself."

"I would, but she insists on having a plastic surgeon."

"Have you tried a goddamned Band Aid?"

"The skin edges are a little uneven and they really do need a couple of stitches to line up the edges of the wound."

Dr. Wisniewski is silent for moment. "All right." he says. "Tell her I'll come in and close it, but my fee will be three hundred dollars. Maybe that will discourage her."

"Three hundred dollars," Miss O'Connor howls. "That is outrageous!" She stares off for a few seconds, and then she asks, "Isn't there a Plastic Surgery *resident* in the hospital?"

How stupid of me. Why hadn't I thought of that? I return to the nurses' station, check the call list, then ask the nurse to page Doctor Whittaker—a first year resident, sleeping in a call room on the fifth floor. He is in the hospital to cover the Burn Unit and any Plastic Surgery patients who need an IV restarted or other routine attention.

I turn to Nikki. "Ask Dr. Whittaker to come down and join us."

After a few minutes, a shiny-faced, bleary-eyed young man comes sauntering into the Emergency Room. He looks all of twenty years old. "Hi there," he says sleepily. "I'm Emory Whittaker, the intern on Plastics." He blinks his eyes under a crown of curly blond hair.

An intern. Probably not much experience. I ask him to join me in a private corner of the Emergency Room.

"What services have you been on?" I ask.

"Anesthesia. And now Plastics."

"Ever closed a wound?"

"A couple times two years ago, when I was a medical student."

"Nothing since?"

"Not yet."

"How about in the lab?"

"Not so far, but I'd like to learn."

It would be so much simpler to just repair the wound myself, but I can't do it without the patient's permission. So off we go to the linen closet to find a clean towel. Then we retreat to the privacy of the call room in the back of the Emergency Room. I cut an "incision" down the center of the towel, and then play the role of teacher. First, I show Dr. Whittaker how to grasp tissues with forceps with his left hand and pass the needle-holder with his right hand.

"Pick up what you're going to sew, but don't crush the tissues."

Then I show him how to rotate the needle-holder to advance the needle through the tissues. "Follow the curve of the rounded needle," I tell him. "Don't just force it through the tissues. And try to align the edges of the wound."

Isn't it remarkable how many detailed steps there are here, and how long it takes to learn them before they become reflexive? God, I must have driven my attending doctors crazy when I was a first year. Maybe I still do.

At first, Dr. Whittaker handles the needle-holder in an awkward fashion. But as he persists, he becomes progressively more skilled.

Then we practice for five minutes tying knots with the suture, laying down the knots in a square, symmetrical fashion.

"Bring the edges of the wound together." I tell him. "But don't make the closure too tight or you'll cut off the blood supply. Wounds need blood to heal."

After fifteen minutes of practice, he seems to be as good as he's going to be in the short time available.

"It's now or never," I say as we march into Miss O'Connor's room.

"Are you the Plastic Surgery resident?" she asks.

"Not really," Dr. Whittaker says sheepishly. "I'm a General Surgery resident, assigned to the Plastic Surgery service for three months."

Assigned to *Plastic Surgery*—the magic words. That's all Miss O'Connor needs to hear.

"Then go ahead," she says.

Dr. Whittaker puts on a mask, and pulls on sterile surgical gloves. Then we drape the wound with sterile towels to expose only the area to be sutured.

"All right, Miss O'Conner," I announce. "Dr. Whitaker is going to inject your skin with Xylocaine, to numb the wound. It's going to burn, but just for a minute or two."

"Okay," she says bravely. "Go ahead, I prefer not to

watch." She turns away to face the wall as Dr. Whittaker begins his repair.

"Dr. Whittaker," I say. "I like the way that you use the forceps in your left hand to lift what you're going to sew."

Dr. Whittaker uses his forceps to lift the skin on one side of the wound.

"And I really like how gentle you are."

Dr. Whittaker grasps the tissues more gently; he relaxes the pinching force he's exerting with the forceps.

"How nicely you rotate your wrist."

Dr. Whittaker stops pushing the needle, and rotates his wrist to follow the curve of the needle.

After he's placed and tied three stitches, the closure appears to be satisfactorily aligned.

He then applies several butterfly strips. Lastly, he peels off his surgical gloves and triumphantly tears off his mask with all the bravura of a man who has just completed his first successful heart transplant. He brushes back his curly blond hair, and we remove the sterile towels and drapes.

Miss O'Connor sits up and inspects her wound. Then she looks up and gives us a radiant smile. "See," she says. "I knew you could find a plastic surgeon for me."

CHAPTER 26

CHEST PAIN

It's eleven o'clock, and I just arrived at the University Emergency Room to begin my eight-hour shift. The resident who was working from three to eleven left early—something about his wife having labor pains. In any case, he's gone, and the ER is mine to worry about. It is as busy as a grocery store the day before Thanksgiving.

A resident on General Surgery and a medical student go rolling past me with a teenage boy on a gurney. They're on their way to the OR.

"Appendicitis," The resident says.

"When I get this place under control, I'll come up to watch you guys do your appendectomy."

"Any time," the resident says.

In Examining Room Two, a Pediatrics resident examines a two-year old child with fever and croup-like cough. The anxious mother hovers protectively over the child, watching the resident's every move.

Alyssa gives me an update about another patient. "Before you got here," she says, "I paged Brofsky, I asked him to come down to see Kasper Crown in Exam Room Three. He's a chronic lunger, on home oxygen, in a wheelchair."

"Where is he now?"

"Outside. Having a smoke."

"On oxygen?"

"He does it all the time. He turns off his oxygen tank for a couple of minutes then lights up and has a few puffs.

"Seems foolhardy to me. One of these days he's going to blow his head off. Either that, or we'll be visiting what's left of him in the Burn Unit."

Brofsky arrives in the ER. "I know Kasper Crown from when he was an inpatient," he says. "He's a *frequent flyer*, in and out of the hospital several times a month. If he makes more than ten ER visits a year, he qualifies for a free flight."

Brofsky starts to laugh. "Too bad for Kasper. He's on Public Aid. All his flights are free. I wonder if he can bequeath the free visits to his children."

"Bubble gum Louis is here." Alyssa says. "He has a patient from the psych facility."

"What's going on here?" I ask Alyssa. "Are we having some kind of reunion or something?"

"No reunion," she says. "It's just that with no doctor here to see the patients and move them along, they start piling up."

"Louis," she says, "Is in Room Four with a new patient named Walton from the psych hospital."

I stop in to see him. Mr. Walton is a forty-year old man who cut his finger on a piece of glass. It appears to be a negligible injury, and when I examine him, I find no damage to the nerves or tendons. We give him a tetanus booster, and cleanse his hand. He doesn't need anything more than a band-aid. I suspect that the real reason he's here is so that the night nurse at the psych hospital can show that the injury was examined by an ER physician and the requisite paperwork was filled out.

"Hey, Doc," Louis says. "Mr. Burns is back in the hospital, but he's not allowed to have any coins."

We both laugh.

Nikki comes in and tells me that there is a Mrs. Gargill in Examining Room Three with a rash on her buttock. I enter the examining room with Nikki. Mrs. Gargill, a 65 year old lady, has a red patchy rash on her left buttock. The eruption consists of small fluid-filled raised areas. Mrs. Cargill tells us that they are associated with severe burning pain. My diagnosis is herpes zoster (shingles). She states that she's had the burning rash in this same area before, and that it usually runs its course over two or three weeks.

"What causes it?" Mrs. Cargill asks.

"Chicken pox virus."

"Really! I haven't had chicken pox since I was five years old."

"Yes, but the virus has been living in the nerve cells in your spinal cord. When it's activated, it causes a rash and inflammation on the skin. We can give you an ointment that you can put on the rash, and a prescription for some tablets that work very well, but you must remember to take a pill every five hours for the next six days."

Mrs. Cargill agrees, and we discharge her from the Emergency Room.

The ER is busy with so many diverse problems, I'm not sure I'm going to get out of here in time to see the appendectomy.

As I leave Mrs. Cargill, an ambulance rolls up to the admitting ramp, and the paramedics deliver a bald, sixty-five year old man, bypassing Yolanda. His name is Max Hoffman. Nikki tells the paramedics to put him in Examining Room One. "Looks like an MI," one of the paramedics says discreetly as they wheel by.

Mr. Hoffman is pale and pasty looking. He takes rapid shallow breaths. Alyssa helps him out of his clothes and into a hospital gown.

"Mr. Hoffman!" Allan Brofsky exclaims as he strides into the examining room. "What are you doing here? Didn't I just see you in clinic two or three days ago?" He greets Mr. Hoffman's wife and adult daughter. The whole family of three seems to be relieved when they see Brofsky's familiar face.

While they are chatting, Alyssa hooks up Mr. Hoffman's EKG to a monitor. It reveals dramatic changes suggestive of an acute coronary occlusion, of insufficient blood flow to the heart muscle. It appears to be a heart attack in progress.

"Mr. Hoffman," Brofsky asks. "Are you having chest pain?"

Mr. Hoffman says *yes*, but he insists that it is not severe.

"I don't want to worry my wife," he says quietly.

"Is it sharp pain or pressure?"

"Pressure."

"Show me where it hurts."

Mr. Hoffman points to his left shoulder and middle of his chest.

"For how long has it been bothering you?"

"The last couple of hours. But only when I exert myself."

"When you exert yourself? Like when you climb stairs?"

Mr. Hoffman nods his head *yes*.

Brofsky looks troubled as he studies the EKG monitor tracking the electrical activity of Mr. Hoffman's heart. We also feel abnormal pulses at Mr. Hoffman's wrist. The large number of these abnormal beats is disconcerting. Brofsky presses his stethoscope against Mr. Hoffman's chest to listen to his heart sounds.

Then he turns to Alyssa with orders. "Let's get a twelve lead EKG, blood gases and cardiac enzymes, an IV line and oxygen by mask and give him a couple of nitros under his tongue."

I take Mr. Hoffman's arm, and search for a suitable vein. I find a large vessel, insert a catheter into it, and tape it firmly in place. Now we have intravenous access permitting us to draw blood and rapidly give medications, if we need to.

While Alyssa gathers the vials, needles and syringes she needs, Mr. Hoffman groans, and rolls his eyes back in his head. At that moment, his EKG tracing becomes an aimless jittery line as his heart fibrillates, the individual heart cells contract wildly, without coordination. His heart now provides no blood flow to his brain, heart muscle or other organs. He has just minutes to live. The EKG alarm screeches a high-pitched alert.

Brofsky rips open Mr. Hoffman's hospital gown and begins to give cardiac massage (CPR). He rhythmically pushes down on his patient's chest. Each push squeezes the heart, causing it to empty blood into Mr. Hoffman's arteries, nourishing the tissues; with each release, it refills with blood returning to the heart from the veins.

Everyone in the room gathers about the gurney except Nikki, who shepherds the Hoffman family to a small chapel adjacent to the Emergency Room, a place of privacy and spiritual solace. It also takes the family away from the staff while we are in the midst of a clinical crisis.

Meanwhile, Alyssa wheels the crash cart into the room. This is a large utility cart, pre-stocked with equipment and medications required to treat a sudden cardiac arrest.

I push my way to the head of the gurney, take an endotracheal tube that Alyssa has ready for me, and try to insert it into Mr. Hoffman's airway. But I cannot see; Mr. Hoffman's mouth and throat are filled with thick mucus and vomitus. Alyssa hands me a suction catheter to clear the field. Now I can see. I insert the endotracheal tube between his vocal cords and in his airway. I'm certain that the tube is located properly in the airway, but I take no chances. I take my stethoscope to check the location of the tube. The breath sounds are normal and are equal on the two sides of his chest; I feel certain that the endotracheal tube is in proper position. I tape it in place.

I connect the tube to a hand-operated Ambu bag, and I rhythmically squeeze the football-like Ambu-bag to ventilate Mr. Hoffman's lungs. I hear an alert for cardiac arrest announced on the public address system—"Code Blue, Emergency Room; Code Blue, Emergency Room." More help will be on the way.

Father Burmeister, the hospital chaplain, pokes his head in the doorway of the examining room with a searching look.

"The family's in the chapel," Alyssa says.

Another medical resident arrives. He takes over the chest compressions. At the same time, Brofsky reaches for the defibrillator on the counter beside the patient. He grips the device's handles, and checks them to be sure the machine is charged. He applies the paddles to Mr. Hoffman's chest and shouts, "Clear." Everyone stops what they are doing, and takes a step back, away from the gurney. Brofsky pushes the red activation button, and this discharges a powerful electric shock through the paddles and through Mr. Hoffman's chest. The shock momentarily lifts Mr. Hoffman up and off the gurney, but it does not reestablish a normal heart rhythm.

Brofsky turns to Alyssa. "One milligram of epinephrine IV. Follow that with 80 of bicarb."

Alyssa is ready. She holds IV syringes filled with appropriate doses of medications that are used to treat cardiac arrests.

This was a *witnessed* cardiac arrest, *witnessed* because it occurred in our presence; therefore, we know exactly how long the heart and brain have been deprived of oxygen-rich blood.

Brofsky applies the defibrillation paddles again and again to defibrillate Mr. Hoffman's heart. He growls under his breath, beseeching the recalcitrant heart to respond.

"Come on," he pleads. "Beat for us, beat for us." He orders a series of drugs to be given in addition to the electrical defibrillation, but nothing is successful—the disorganized tracings of ventricular fibrillation persist. Just a short time ago, Max Hoffman was talking to us, denying substantial chest pain; now we are attempting to save the same unconscious person who has not had a normal heartbeat in more than half an hour.

Brofsky seems unshakeable in his commitment. "Come on, come on." His tone changes to that of a supplicant. But there is no response. Finally, after forty-five minutes, Brofsky reluctantly calls a halt to the resuscitation effort, and sits dejectedly on a stainless steel stool.

He is exhausted. "I hate to quit," he says apologetically to the dead man whom he knew.

After a painful moment of introspection, Brofsky rises and motions to me to join him. "Let's go talk to the family," he says. Neither of us relishes the idea of facing them alone.

We see Mrs. Hoffman and her daughter in the chapel, and I can tell by their faces that they know what we are about to say.

Mrs. Hoffman collapses onto a couch the moment we speak, first screaming, and then wailing uncontrollably. Her daughter rushes to console her, but she is as sorrow-stricken as her mother.

"How could this be?" Mrs. Hoffman asks. "He was awake and talking to us when we came in."

"It was his heart," Brofsky explains. "We gave him dozens of electric shocks, and all kinds of cardiac medications, but nothing would bring his heart back. We think it was a massive heart attack."

"Can we see him?" the daughter asks.

"Yes, of course. Just as soon as Nikki and Alyssa get the room in order."

Mrs. Hoffman is overcome with sorrow. Father Burmeister does his best to console her, but there is little that anyone can say or do. An hour ago, Mr. Hoffman was alive and speaking to us; now he is gone. The unexpected shock of his loss is as powerful as the loss itself. Moreover, soon the family will have to make funeral arrangements, an action that will confirm the undeniable reality of it all.

Alyssa appears in the chapel doorway. "Mrs. Hoffman," she says with a kindness I have never heard from her before. "You can come in and be with Mr. Hoffman now. Alyssa and Father Burmeister lead the Hoffmans into the now-tidy examining room, and they promptly leave the family with Mr. Hoffman.

Brofsky and I remain in the corridor, physically exhausted and emotionally drained. Without warning, there is a shriek as Mr. Hoffman's daughter comes running out of the examining room. "He's not dead." She screams. "He moved. I saw it myself. I'm sure of it."

Brofsky and I join the family in the examining room and check Mr. Hoffman. I touch his skin; his body is beginning to cool. I reconnect his EKG to the wall-mounted display. There is an obvious signal sweeping across the screen when I hold the EKG leads in my hands, but there is none when the leads are attached to Mr. Hoffman. I call the Hoffman family's attention to his chest. There are no signs of spontaneous respirations.

"Those are just agonal reflexes," Brofsky says.

"Agony?" Mrs. Hoffman asks with alarm.

"Not agony, Mrs. Hoffman. *Agonal.* Reflex movements that remain for a time after a person has passed on. Believe me, Mrs. Hoffman. Your husband has passed on; his body is getting cold. He really cannot feel pain." How could he? His brain has not been perfused with oxygenated blood for about an hour, far longer than the critical three to five minutes.

Another hour slips by before the Hoffmans, with Reverend Burmeister's help, gather sufficient strength to call a funeral home. I return to the other end of the Emergency Room corridor to my little call room bed where I wait for the nighttime hours to pass. I am too agitated to sleep.

CHAPTER 27

NIGHT MUSIC

Tonight will be my last night of moonlighting, my swan song in the Emergency Room. And what a night it is.

"Bitter cold," the weatherman warns on the eleven o'clock news. "Ten below zero downtown. Fifteen below in the suburbs. Stay at home if at all possible. And if you must go out, be sure to bundle up."

I couldn't agree more, but I'm not going anywhere. I'll be here from eleven to seven. Maybe this weather will keep the patients at home and I'll be able to get some sleep, but I'm not counting on it. I figure that anyone who bothers to come out on a night like this must have something seriously wrong with them. We may also get some of the homeless from under the viaducts, complete with frostbitten fingers and toes.

It's midnight, and not a single patient has come in yet. Nikki's here, but Alyssa called in to say that her car won't start. I don't doubt it. Mine sounded like a coffee grinder when I cranked it over.

I withdraw to my call room in the back of the ER to read a surgical journal. I'll sit in here until the lure of the bed in the call room is more than I can resist. But the cold is relentless. It seeps right through the walls, gnaws at my arms and legs under my thin cotton scrubs. There are some blankets on the bed, but they're skimpy polyester things, and aren't thick enough to do much good. I turn off the light, pull the blankets up under my chin and try to sleep.

Twelve-thirty, I'm still awake when one of the hospital guards makes his hourly walk-through. He's singing *Ol' Man River*, and his robust baritone voice comes booming around the corner well before he does. If I were up seeing patients, I wouldn't even notice him, but listening to him while I'm trying to sleep is another matter. I suspect his singing is especially irritating to patients who are dozing, waiting for their x-rays or lab results to come back.

There is a pair of pneumatically-operated glass doors that leads out of the ER and onto the ambulance drop-off ramp. They hiss-thump each time the doors swing open. Hiss-thump, hiss-thump, a signal that someone is coming in or going out, or that one of the staff is cutting through the ER to the main hospital. Or it may be one of the guards making his hourly rounds. Whoever it is, every opening of the doors is accompanied by a hiss-thump, hiss-thump and, a moment later, by an icy blast that races down the Emergency Room corridor to bite my skin.

I get up and raid the ER linen closet for four more of those doilies they call blankets. The double doors have an opaque layer of ice on them, and someone has laid towels on the floor to catch the water dripping down. But it's too cold for much of it to melt. Nikki sits in the nurses' station, wrapped head to toe in a tan blanket, looking for all the world like a tee-pee.

"What are you doing?" I ask.

"What do you think I'm doing?" She snaps. "Trying to keep warm."

"Why is it so cold down here?"

"Because the heat comes out of those stupid ceiling vents instead of vents near the floor. And of course, those doors opening every few minutes doesn't help any."

Poor Nikki. I can hide in the call room, but she's got to sit out there and take it until seven a.m.

There's a radio in the nurses' station that's part of a network that ties together all the ambulances with all the hospital ER's in the area. Crackling, mechanical-sounding voices chatter constantly announcing that an ambulance is en route with a patient to one hospital or another. And the target hospitals answer back, their acknowledgements punctuated with as many *ten-fours* as the staff can cram into a call. Everyone seems to think they are on television. The constant babble is relentless, but one can't just ignore it because sooner or later, one of those ambulances will be headed in our direction. Right now, there's no one aiming for us. I go back to bed and try to sleep or, at the very least, to keep warm.

Must be one a.m. because here comes Ernie with the linen cart, squeaking and thumping as it rolls past my door. It sounds like it has a fluttering wheel, or maybe one that grabs now and then. Whatever it is, it's been doing it for months, and no one has bothered to fix it. It's especially annoying tonight.

"Hey mon, how's eva-buddy doin'?" Ernie calls out with his exaggerated Jamaican patois. Someone told me he's really from the Bronx. "Here's what you been waiting for, more sheets and pillow cases. The hospital's clean out of blankets."

Hiss-thump, hiss-thump. It's one-thirty. I recognize Father Burmeister's voice and his hurried steps as he passes the nurses' station. "How are you doing, Nikki?" he asks. "Can't stop now. Got to go to the ICU."

Someone must be in trouble up there.

It's now two a.m. Bottles clinking and banging on a rattling cart. It's Harlan from Pharmacy replenishing the ER's stock of IV fluids and medications. This is his usual drop-off time.

"Eva-buddy doin' okay?" he asks. "Cold enough for you?"

Still, not a single patient.

Yolanda, the dark-haired woman who works at the reception desk, and Nikki have gotten into a noisy conversation, and I hear them as clearly as if they were

215

standing right outside my call room door. Whatever they're talking about must be hilarious. Now Nikki is carrying on about some movie she saw.

Hiss-thump. Hiss-thump. Three a.m. It's Simone from Admitting. She often takes a shortcut across the parking lot to bring us a copy of the midnight census. It lets us know which floors have empty beds available. With so many people unable to start their cars and get into work, I hope we'll have the staff to cover all our patients.

Simone likes to stop and visit with the ER staff. Nikki and Yolanda are probably all talked out by now; I'll bet they're ready for some new company.

Hiss-thump, hiss-thump. Four a.m. It's time for Mrs. Greer, the Night Nursing Supervisor, to make her rounds. She's a classy, soft-spoken lady who runs the hospital between 11 p.m. and 7 a.m. Her job is to move nursing staff around to where they are needed.

The regular night crew—Nikki and B.J., Yolanda, Ernie and Harlan, Simone, Mrs. Greer, the guards, the regular floor nurses, and people I don't even know—work here every night from eleven to seven. They are here to finish up yesterday's work, and prepare for tomorrow.

Hiss-thump, hiss-thump. Five a.m. and I'm still awake. Sounds like a party out there. I drag myself out to have a look. It's the county police visiting the ER for a warm up and to mooch some hot coffee. I'll bet they brought doughnuts. They're policemen; they always bring doughnuts. They love to hang around the ER. Policemen seem to be especially fond of our nurses—clean and starched white, not like the grimy world they regularly face.

Yolanda and Nikki are perched on stools in the nurses' station, wrapped in tan blankets. They're surrounded by a platoon of burly cops in black leather jackets, performing for the girls. One of the cops can't take his eyes off Yolanda. He tells her that on this frigid night she looks like a "hundred-pound Popsicle." That gets a big laugh.

I visit with the county's finest for a while and laugh at their wisecracks. I've been known to drive a little too fast on occasion, and I would like it if these folks recognized me if they stop me. After all, we night people are in this together. After a few minutes of listening to their lame jokes, I head back to the call room, slip under the mountain of polyester blankets and return to the night music of the hospital.

Six forty-five a.m. I've finally drifted off to sleep when one of the day shift residents comes crashing into the call room and flips on the lights. He towers over me like a giant dressed in a puffy down-filled parka that makes him look like the Michelin Tire man. His hood is up, and he's puffing steam in the cold call room.

"Sorry to wake you," he says. "You must have had a busy night."

"Not really," I tell him. "We didn't have a single patient come in last night."

"Really! So you must have had a good night's sleep."

PHILIP B. DOBRIN, M.D.

CHAPTER 28

AORTIC ANEURYSMS

I am about to begin a three month rotation on Vascular Surgery, a rotation I've been looking forward to. The attending doctors on that service do a large number of diagnostic and therapeutic procedures, and I am eager to learn to do them also.

***

Dr. Benton is the Chief of Vascular Surgery at University Hospital. The residents who have worked with him say he is an outstanding technical surgeon, a fine teacher, and that he has a thorough understanding of the current controversies in vascular surgery. In many ways, Dr. Benton is a man from whom an ambitious resident has much to learn.

On Monday evening, Dr. Benton asks me to come to his office to discuss two of our patients.

"We have two patients with abdominal aortic aneurysms," he says, "Mr. Snow and Mr. Twitchel. Both men are in their sixties, and both have aortic aneurysms that are six centimeters in diameter. That size puts both of them at high risk for spontaneous rupture of the aneurysm."

I think of Mr. Hall, the gentlemen whom I met when I was a first year resident. Mr. Hall had a small aortic aneurysm and also a possible hernia. We admitted him for a workup, but we were shocked when he died during the night from leaking of his aneurysm. The small size of the aneurysm shows how hazardous even a small one can be.

"Unexpectedly," Benton continues, "some OR time has become available tomorrow, and I will be available as well; so I plan to operate on both patients, one right after the other. How about you give me a hand in the OR?"

"Yes, of course," I say politely. Actually, I'm thrilled—a big-time case and for the first time I will be operating with Dr. Benton, a specialist in vascular surgery.

"Here's the plan," Benton says." "I'll do Snow, and you scrub and be my first assistant. Then we will do Twitchel, but we'll switch roles; you'll do the case, and I'll be your first assistant."

This sounds perfect, an ideal way to learn to do aneurysm surgery—by serving as an apprentice to an expert. I'll be able to follow every step performed by Dr. Benton on Mr. Snow, and utilize the same techniques on Mr. Twitchel. Tonight I intend to review everything I can regarding the surgery of abdominal aortic aneurysms.

***

We start morning rounds at six-thirty and are finished by seven o'clock. I leave the group to join Dr. Benton in the operating room.

Our first case is Mr. Snow. We pass a few pleasantries with him before the anesthesiologists put him to sleep. When he is anesthetized, we scrub, gown and glove as usual. We gather at the OR table and watch Dr. Benton make a longitudinal incision in the midline. Once we have entered the abdomen, he finds no pathology that would preclude the planned aneurysm surgery.

The aorta is the largest artery in the body, and it carries blood from the heart to virtually all the diverse organs. We identify the bulging, aneurysmally-dilated aorta, and cross clamp it just above and just below the aneurysm. I can't take my eyes off that damned aneurysm.

A sudden tear in that artery wall would be the end of all things for Mr. Snow, like a fire hose emptying its contents in just a drenching second or two. No, I am not touching anything near that vessel.

Dr. Benton takes special care to not disturb the aneurysm or damage the renal arteries. These vessels come off the aorta high, usually above the location where one finds an aortic aneurysm. The renal arteries are critically important because they deliver blood to the kidneys. Without them, a patient would require dialysis to clear the urine of the waste products of metabolism.

Dr. Benton now focuses on the aneurysm. With the artery clamped above and below the lesion, he takes a scalpel and carefully opens the aneurysmal aorta. Then he inserts a tubular Dacron graft into the lumen of the opened aneurysmal aorta. It looks like one cylinder placed within another. In fact, that's exactly what it is. He sews the top end of the cylindrical Dacron graft to the aorta *above* the aneurysm, and he sews the bottom end of the Dacron graft to the aorta *below* the aneurysm. Dr. Benton uses tough non-absorbable stitches to sew the Dacron graft to the thin shell of remaining aneurysmal aorta. Sewing these tissues together gives them increased strength.

When the cross clamps are removed, blood flows from the above, through the tubular graft, and into all the body's other organs. Finally, he closes what is left of the aneurysmal shell that has been the aorta around the tubular graft. He does this to separate the operated aorta from the nearby loops of bowel, which otherwise might erode into the graft.

Three hours after we began, everything looks like that depicted in the Vascular Surgery textbooks, neat and anatomically correct. Mr. Snow awakens from the operation in the Post Anesthesia Care Unit with a strengthened aorta, and normal renal function. Documentation of his urinary output every ten or fifteen minutes during the operation by the anesthesiologists shows that he is producing a satisfactory thirty milliliters per hour of urine throughout the case.

We sit for a few minutes in the doctors' lounge, resting our tension-stressed feet and aching backs. Hey, this surgery isn't so difficult! I can learn to do it. I've learned a lot already, but it's risky, and one must not make a mistake; everything happens fast.

***

Our second patient is Mr.Twitchel, a burly gentleman who owns an ice cream parlor and, it appears, frequently samples his wares. He also has a six centimeter abdominal aortic aneurysm. We use the same surgical approach as we did for Mr. Snow, but this time, *I* am the primary surgeon. Dr. Benton hovers over me like a protective parent, intervening and directing me whenever I stumble.

As Dr. Benton did with Mr. Snow, we open the abdomen using a midline incision. After examining the abdominal organs, we apply clamps across the abdominal aorta above and below the aneurysm. I am certainly more hesitant than Dr. Benton was with Mr. Snow, but he is a patient teacher.

Now I make a longitudinal incision to open the aorta for the length of the aneurysm. And, as Dr. Benton did when operating on Mr. Snow, I place a tubular Dacron graft in the lumen of the aneurysmal aorta. The tubular graft will support the thin aortic wall and will act as a conduit for blood flow. As with Mr. Snow, the opened aneurysm appears as one cylindrical structure within another. The anesthesiologists assure us that Mr. Twitchel's pulse and blood pressure are stable, and that he is making a satisfactory volume of urine.

Then, repeating Dr. Benton's steps, I sew the proximal end of the Dacron graft to the aorta above the aneurysm, and sew the distal end of the tubular Dacron graft to the aorta below the aneurysm. So far, everything I'm doing replicates what Dr. Benton did in Mr. Snow. But all at once everything changes; we are shocked to discover that Mr. Twitchel's aorta is too fragile to hold stitches. His atherosclerosis-clogged artery resembles a tube filled with crumbling cottage cheese. The tough stitches cut through the flimsy artery wall.

Without hesitation, Dr. Benton takes over the operation, and I stand paralyzed, uncertain as to what to do. Help, I tell myself; give him exposure, but stay out of his way. Three times Dr. Benton tries to sew the Dacron graft to the aorta with the tough non-absorbable stitches, but each time they cut effortlessly through the wall of the artery. Dr. Benton has no choice but to reposition the cross clamps higher and higher, until he is clamping across the renal arteries. This impedes renal blood flow. Clamping these arteries must be for just a few minutes or the kidneys will be injured and the patient will be banished to a world of dialysis three times per week.

Finally, there is good news. At this high location, the aortic tissue is stronger than it is more distally. Benton's stitches hold and we are able to remove the vascular clamps. Benton expeditiously completes the operation. What had begun as a demonstration of routine surgical technique had become a dangerous challenge. Thank goodness Benton was skilled and was standing beside me.

***

We sit in a circle in the Surgical ICU, Dr. Benton, a medical student and I, staring at Mr. Twitchel, as though our most salubrious thoughts could somehow drive out all the insufficiencies of that fragile aorta.

"What about Morbidity and Mortality (M and M) Conference," the medical student asks? "Do we have to report it?"

"Report what?" Dr. Benton snaps. "We came upon anatomic changes we didn't expect. We modified our surgical procedure, and, so far, we seem to have made the right decisions. We don't have to present this case at M and M for doing the *right* thing."

It is a sobering lesson, as with everything in surgery: if you do enough procedures in enough patients you will encounter lots of good results, and every kind of unwelcome surprise."

But an aortic wall that is too fragile to hold stitches—I never would have expected it. And, apparently

Dr. Benton didn't expect it either. I make a mental note to print an entry on one of my trusty three-by-five cards— Mr. Twitchel, Check lab values three times a week. And while I'm at it I'd better call the renal service, the Internal Medicine doctors who specialize in kidney failure. Just in case.

CHAPTER 29

SENIOR YEAR ORIENTATION

Tomorrow Lenny and I will enter the senior year of our residency. Dr. Peterson invites the two of us to visit him in his office. *Senior orientation,* he calls it. We go, of course, and sit outside his office waiting. Even though there is no moon-like clock on the wall, we are not one second late.

Peterson's office consists of a small desk with an extensive surgical library that covers one entire wall, floor to ceiling. Every book is concerned with medical or scientific issues, but even more remarkable is the fact that most of the data and wisdom cited in those books have been incorporated into Peterson's personal memory. I have heard him quote risks, advantages, and mortalities of different treatments and procedures used for various medical indications. How does he keep all that information in his head? By necessity, I suppose. As Peterson says, "You must know the data if you are going to recommend one or another treatment to a patient."

A radio or cassette player sits hidden on a shelf somewhere in his closet-like office. As might be expected, the room is bathed in the music of Bach.

"Do you ever listen to anything besides Bach?" I ask him.

"Like whom?

"Like Mozart or Beethoven."

"Mozart? Beethoven?" Peterson shrinks in mock horror. "No," he says. "I don't care for modern music."

"Who is the pianist playing the Bach?" I ask.

"Glenn Gould or Alfred Brendel," Peterson answers.

"I should have known you'd admire Gould and Brendel—the expertise, the precision. . . ."

Peterson nods. "Sometimes I think I'd give up surgery if I could play the piano like Gould or Brendel."

So we all have our heroes; even *our* hero does.

Returning to his personal library, Peterson makes a thoughtful offer. "You can come in here and help yourself to these books any time you need them, whether I'm here or not. But be sure to sign a three-by-five card and leave it in place of the book you borrow so I know where to find it. Books have a way of walking away and not coming back."

We nod appreciatively.

"Now, about the senior year," Peterson says. "There will be two General Surgery Services. You will be the senior on *Service One*," he says pointing to me. "And Lenny will be the senior on *Service Two.*"

"You and Lenny will be more independent than you've been used to, but if you encounter a patient in the middle of the night with an obscure illness don't call me expecting me to make a diagnosis for you over the phone; you call me when you've figured it out and are ready to give me *your* diagnosis."

Seems fair enough.

He turns to me. "Starting tomorrow, you will have Art Mortiz, a fourth year as your junior resident. Do you know him?"

"Yes. An ex-athlete, a good doctor."

"That's him. And pay attention to what he has to say. He has a lot of experience. You two can learn from each other.

"You'll also have Chris Gabel, a first year resident. He has high energy and is voluble. You'll have to keep him focused and the lid on."

"Got it." I make a note to myself to look up the word *voluble*.

226

CHAPTER 30

A LADY WITH ABDOMINAL PAIN

This is the first night of my senior year. It is two o'clock in the morning, and I am awakened by a telephone call from Art Mortiz, the fourth year resident on our service.

"I'm in the Emergency Room," he says, "Seeing a Mrs. D'Annunzio. She's a forty-five year old lady with nausea, vomiting and severe abdominal pain. Her temperature and white blood cell count are slightly elevated. Her EKG is normal."

It would be hazardous to judge this patient's condition from a telephone conversation, so I dress and drive into the ER to see her for myself.

Mrs. D'Annunzio is a mildly obese lady, lying on a gurney, tearfully clutching her bed sheet with a blanched fist. This woman's discomfort is impressive, and I can see why the ER called for a surgical consult. She is accompanied by her three adult daughters and her 75-year old mother, Celeste Lazarra, the irrepressible proprietor of the popular *Italian Market* restaurant.

"Where does it hurt?" I ask Mrs. D'Annunzio.

"Everywhere," she says through clenched teeth. She waves her hand vaguely over her belly.

I rest my stethoscope on her abdomen and listen for bowel sounds, the rumbling, gurgling signature of gas and liquids passing through the intestines. These sounds often are subdued or absent in patients with serious intra-abdominal pathology. In Mrs. D'Annunzio, her bowel sounds are normal.

I rest my palm against her abdomen and gradually apply pressure. She tolerates this without complaint. Then, without warning, I abruptly withdraw my hand. Pain elicited by this sudden maneuver is called *rebound tenderness*, and is a sign of inflammation of the peritoneum, i.e. the film-like sac that surrounds the intestines. But Mrs. D'Annunzio has no rebound tenderness.

So, she has severe abdominal pain without rebound tenderness, a slight fever, and no obvious diagnosis. I can hear Dr. Peterson's exhortation now—"Don't call me in the middle of the night with a list of symptoms and expect me to figure out what's wrong with your patient; make a diagnosis *before* you call me." After examining her I stand in the hall outside her room, mulling over my findings. Whatever is wrong with this lady, the severity of her symptoms is impressive.

Over the past four years of residency, I've made some personal observations about how we arrive at a diagnosis. In about seventy-five or eighty percent of patients, we are guided by the medical history, i.e., what the patient tells us. That doesn't help much here as Mrs. D'Annunzio has vague ill-defined pain and no proven medical history. In about fifteen percent of patients we make a diagnosis based on what we find on physical examination. In the remaining ten percent of patients we make a diagnosis based on laboratory results or x-ray findings. Often we use these tests to *confirm* a presumptive diagnosis. But in Mrs. D'Annunzio's case, we have no presumptive diagnosis.

Art and I leave Mrs. D'Annunzio to retreat to the nurses' station to talk this over. Almost unnoticed, Celeste Lazarra, Mrs. D'Annunzio's mother, comes padding along beside us in her stocking feet.

"Why don't you wait here with your daughter?" I ask. "We'll be out in just a minute."

"Oh, no," she says. ""I want to hear what-a-you say."

"Could be food poisoning," Art suggests. "She's had some nausea and vomiting, but no diarrhea."

"Can't be food poisoning," Mrs. Lazarra says indignantly. "The only food she eat was in our restaurant—melanzana—eggplant, baked in a hot oven. We have a clean-a kitchen. She doesn't get sick from *my* kitchen."

Art puts an x-ray film of Mrs. D'Annunzio's abdomen on the wall-mounted illuminated view box. We examine it for diagnostic clues. There is no evidence of free air as would be present if there were perforation of the stomach or bowel. There is no evidence of bowel obstruction. Mrs. Lazarra peers at the film as well, her untrained eyes surveying the abstract black and gray images.

"What's-a-this?" she asks, pointing to a curved structure.

"That's the lung," I tell her.

"Ah-ha," she says thoughtfully.

"And this?"

"That's the diaphragm."

"I see," she says. She is an apt pupil. Educated or not, she exhibits an essential characteristic—curiosity.

Art points to a normal pattern of gas and stool. The film doesn't show anything abnormal.

We review the results of the laboratory tests—blood work and urinalysis.

Mrs. Lazarra looks over our shoulder. "Are they bad, these tests?"

"No," I tell her. "There is a suggestion of inflammation, but no evidence of pancreatitis."

Mrs. Lazarra nods her head in passive agreement. I'm sure she hasn't the slightest idea of what I'm talking about.

After a few minutes, Art and I return to Mrs. D'Annunzio. Again, Mrs. Lazarra follows along with us. To our surprise, we find Mrs. D'Annunzio sitting up on the gurney, with a hint of a smile. Her debilitating pain is nearly gone. Art and I are taken aback by her clinical improvement. What could have been the source of her severe discomfort? And where has it gone?

I ask Nikki to join me in the examining room, and I ask everyone else to wait outside in the hall. Then I examine Mrs. D'Annunzio again. This time I include a rectal exam, a pelvic exam, and a thorough abdominal examination, but I find nothing abnormal. Now I have no reason to admit her to the hospital, but I'm still puzzled by what caused her symptoms. I decide to keep her in the Emergency Room for a few hours to follow her progress.

It's too late to drive all the way home and back again for morning rounds, so I go up to the fifth floor resident's quarters to find an unoccupied call room. Thirty minutes later Nikki calls to tell me that Mrs. D'Annunzio's pain has returned. I hurry back to the ER to see Mrs. D'Annunzio. She is with her three daughters and Mrs. Lazarra.

"Where does it hurt?" I ask the patient. "Where is it most painful? Try to point to *exactly* where it hurts."

She points to the right upper quadrant of her abdomen, to just below her ribs, directly over her gall bladder. Now we have a likely diagnosis—biliary colic, i.e., pain that comes and goes, possibly cholecystitis, i.e., inflammation of the gall bladder, most likely caused by gall stones. Moreover, the changes in her laboratory values are consistent with that diagnosis. I explain all this to Mrs. D'Annunzio, Mrs. Lazarra, and Mrs. D'Annunzio's three daughters.

"We are going to need an ultrasound test," I say. "To see if you have stones in your gall bladder. We are going to give you some mild pain medicine and send you home now, but you must avoid eating large meals, and you must stay away from fatty foods."

Mrs. D'Annunzio, Mrs. Lazarra and the Society of Concerned Daughters all nod their heads in unison.

"We'll call you in the morning to let you know when the ultrasound test is scheduled."

Mrs. D'Annunzio and her family are smiling, pleased that we have a likely explanation for her pain. How dumb of me to not have considered cholecystitis (inflammation of the gall bladder) and cholelithiasis (gall stones) as likely diagnoses. Privately I chastise myself for not considering them sooner. It's four a.m. Perhaps now we can all get some sleep.

***

It is 6:30 a.m.; the morning sun is shining in through the call room window. Heaven only knows how many nights I've slept in this room, or *tried* to sleep, over the past four years, but in the past I've always been a lineman following directions; now I'm a quarterback calling the signals.

I gather our team and we begin rounds. We have just a few patients left for us by the previous service, all post-op and ready for discharge. Flush with a likely diagnosis of Mrs. D'Annunzio's mysterious illness, we wander over to the cafeteria for coffee and breakfast. While sitting there, I take the opportunity to bestow some wisdom on our students.

"She fits the textbook stereotype perfectly for a patient with gall stone disease," I say. "Remember the seven F's mnemonic: *Fair, Female, Forty, Fat, Flabby, Fertile and Flatulent*. Actually, you don't need all seven clues; just the first four will do."

Don't I sound smart? Well, I think to myself, if I'm so smart, why didn't I think of gall stone disease *before* she pointed to her gall bladder? Maybe that's why the residency takes five years. You have to see everything at least once and more often than that; of course, not every abdominal pain is gall bladder disease.

At eight-thirty, Art Mortiz gets on the phone to schedule an ultrasound study of the gall bladder for Mrs. D'Annunzio. She's on for Tuesday morning. We'll call her later in the morning to inform her, after she's had a few hours of sleep. If the ultrasound test shows gallstones, we'll schedule her for a visit to Dr. Peterson's clinic. If she has symptomatic gallstones, we really should remove her gall bladder.

I'm looking forward to seeing Dr. Peterson this morning and telling him about our middle of the night puzzle. He strolls into the cafeteria at eight-thirty, and I start to relate the story to him. But before I get halfway through the story, he interrupts me.

"Sounds to me like biliary colic, right upper quadrant pain that comes and goes. Maybe cholecystitis. You need an ultrasound of the gall bladder in that lady."

"Yes, of course, I do," I say. But before I finish my story he turns and walks away.

Why do I feel like I'm talking to Lenny Goldstein?

***

It's been a week since we saw Mrs. D'Annunzio in the Emergency Room. The ultrasound examination showed that she does, in fact, have stones in her gall bladder, with no suggestion of stones in the common duct. She also has no medical history suggestive on stones in the ducts. Following her ultrasound test, we schedule her to see Dr. Peterson in clinic. After reviewing her history, the ultrasound test results and examination, Peterson recommends that her gall bladder be surgically removed. After some hesitation she agrees, and we'll be doing her surgery next week.

CHAPTER 31

SURGICAL REMOVAL OF GALL BLADDER

We scrub our hands and forearms at the sink outside the operating room, preparing to remove Mrs. D'Annunzio's gall bladder. Our patient lies anesthetized on the operating table under the watchful eyes of Dr. Chung and an Anesthesia resident. Dr. Chung administers the preoperative antibiotics we ordered. We're giving them as a precaution as we will be opening the biliary system which may harbor bacteria in the bile. Antibiotics must be given 60-90 minutes *before* we make the incision in order to be effective. If we wait until after we opened the biliary tract, or until after surgery, antibiotics would provide little if any benefit. We learned these principles from objective, controlled clinical studies.

Internal medicine doctors tend to think of surgeons as being solely concerned with technical matters—anatomy, cutting and sewing of tissue. But there is so much more to surgical science: the indications and timing of operations, the complications of surgery and how we can avoid and treat them and the use and misuse of antibiotics. There is so much emerging information.

While we scrub, Dr. Peterson gives the students a quick review of gall bladder disease. He loves to teach; you can hear it in his voice. And the students value every word of it.

"We need bile to digest fats," he says. "The liver manufactures bile and the gall bladder stores it, acting like a holding tank. When we eat a fatty meal, the gall bladder contracts, expelling bile through the cystic duct, into the common duct, and on into the intestine where it helps with digestion.

"Unfortunately for chemical reasons, some people form stones in their bile; when the gall bladder in these people contracts, the stones can block the outflow to the cystic duct, and this causes painful distention of the gall bladder. That's probably what caused Mrs. D'Annunzio's pain, and that's why we're removing her gall bladder.

"Why not just open the gall bladder?" Veronica asks. "Take out the stones and leave the gall bladder in?"

"We could," Peterson says. "But the gall bladder often is inflamed and might leak post-operatively. It also is likely to form new stones."

He glances at the clock. "Enough talk, time to go to work." He drops his scrub brush in the sink and we march into the operating room.

Today will be my first gall bladder operation as a senior resident. I've been here many times before as a junior resident, but this is the real thing. I know what I'm doing. I'm feeling confident. I make a sharply-defined incision in the skin, an "oblique" cut that runs parallel to the lower edge of the right rib cage. We control skin and muscle bleeding with pressure and stitches, and by using electrocautery, a hand-held pencil-like device that passes electric current through bleeding tissue causing it to coagulate. Peterson and I clamp and cut superficial muscles, and we enter the abdomen.

The students stare wide-eyed at the sight before them. Unlike their experiences in Anatomy class where they studied cadavers, this is their first opportunity to see intra-abdominal structures in a living person, the organs shifting slightly to and fro with each breath.

Each abdominal organ lies in its prescribed place, like sweaters and shirts folded and tucked neatly in a dresser drawer. Some of the organs are readily visible, but others overlap and are partly concealed by other organs. Our first task is to assess, by vision and palpation, each organ in the abdomen. Before we operate on the gall bladder; we must be certain that there are no other unsuspected diseases of the stomach, intestine, liver or spleen. If there were and we did not identify it, we would be rewarded by an unpleasant visit to Dr. Quinn's Morbidity and Mortality (M and M) Conference.

I reach my gloved hand into the abdominal cavity and feel the stomach and its junction with the esophagus. Deep behind the stomach and beneath the diaphragm, my fingers must assess what my eyes cannot see. The esophagus and stomach feel normal. Then I proceed clockwise around the abdomen to evaluate the large and small intestine, the spleen and kidneys. I am especially careful to not injure or tear the fragile spleen. All these structures look and feel normal. While I am in this region, I check for an unsuspected aortic aneurysm; there is none. I continue clockwise until I've examined all the abdominal organs including those that I can reach in the pelvis. I can see and feel the appendix; it appears to be normal. The ovaries cannot be felt: a normal condition for a postmenopausal woman. Finally, my survey brings me back to the liver and gall bladder.

I see and feel no tumors or masses of the liver, gall bladder or pancreas. I cannot feel Mrs. D'Annunzio's biliary stones, but that is not surprising; according to the ultrasound, they are small about the size tomato seeds or perhaps a little larger. Next, I examine and feel the first part of the small intestine and the pancreas.

Dr. Peterson repeats my examination, survey of the abdomen, and he agrees with my assessment. That completed, we are ready to do the operation we came for, a cholecystectomy, i.e., removal of the stone-ladened gall bladder. I grasp the tip of the gall bladder with a clamp, and carefully dissect it free of surrounding fat and connective tissue. We control bleeding as we progress. I am especially careful to not injure the common duct. This region of the body is fraught with anatomic variations.

The key structures must be identified in the crowded space between the liver, gall bladder and the small intestine. Tying off the wrong artery or injuring the common duct could be disastrous. Identification is accomplished by examination and meticulous dissection. Dr. Peterson is a master of it, and he accomplishes it so subtly that often the resident believes that it is he, not Peterson, who is doing it.

We use hemostats and the electrocautery to control bleeding. We also use absorbent white sterile towels called laparotomy pads (*lap pads*) to apply pressure to control bleeding. These pads have a large stainless steel ring attached to them to help us see them on x-ray. The identifying rings are essential because, after lap pads are soaked with blood, they are nearly indistinguishable from oozing dissected living tissues.

Throughout this, and every other operation, the circulating nurse counts every lap pad, surgical needle and instrument that we use. She lays each item on a table beside the operating table after it has been used. She must be sure that each item we use is removed from the patient. At the end of the operation, before we close the abdomen, the number of lap pads, needles and instruments we used *must* match the number counted at the beginning of the operation. If they do not, we must search in the open abdomen to find what is missing. At the same time, the circulating nurse rolls a magnetic roller on the operating room floor to find any curved surgical needles that might have fallen and bounced away. If all these maneuvers fail to retrieve a missing item, we will take an x-ray picture in the operating room with the abdomen still open; we must find the missing item.

After we remove the gall bladder, we inject a few milliliters of radio-opaque contrast material into the cystic duct and common duct to obtain an x-ray picture. This reveals that there are no residual stones in the cystic duct or common duct. If we had identified any remaining stones, we would have had to open those ducts and remove the stones. Finally, Peterson asks the medical students to use some surgical instruments on the excised gall bladder on a table beside the operating table. He wants them to open the gall bladder and identify the presence of small gall stones. There they are!

We are nearly finished. The circulating nurse tells us that our lap pad, needle and instrument counts match our beginning numbers. We wash out the abdomen with sterile saline, and then begin our closure. We use large diameter, absorbable stitches. These will take about six weeks to dissolve. That is the approximate time required for the healing wound to restore most of its native strength.

Remarkably, an hour and twenty minutes has flashed by. There simply is no activity that grips one's attention like performing surgery.

After we close the abdominal incision, Dr. Chung terminates anesthesia, and our focus shifts from the anatomy, surgery and control of bleeding to Mrs. D'Annunzio's ability to breathe on her own. When she is awake and able to breath, Dr. Chung removes the endotracheal breathing tube from her airway. Then we slide her onto a gurney brought up beside the operating table, and we wheel her into the post anesthesia recovery room (PAR). Dr. Chung says something to me about the operation. I can tell he's pleased because he's smiling and waving his arms, but as usual, I really cannot understand him.

In the PAR, Art writes post-op orders for IV fluids and post-op pain medications. After abdominal surgery, patients tend to take small, shallow breaths to avoid pulling painfully on their incision. But taking shallow breaths increases the risk of accumulating mucous secretions in their lungs and developing pneumonia. We will help Mrs. D'Annunzio to take deep breaths by teaching her to put a pillow against her chest and abdomen when she inhales and coughs. We also encourage her to use a plastic incentive spirometer device. Shades of Mr. Cook come to mind. When I was a first year resident Barney assigned me the task of getting Mr. Cook to take

PHILIP B. DOBRIN, M.D.

deep breaths as he was recovering from his large bowel resection. I direct Veronica, our medical student, with a similar responsibility for assisting Mrs. D'Annunzio.

While Art writes post-op orders, I dictate the operative report. It is a detailed step-by-step description of what we did and what we found during the operation. In case there is an untoward outcome, the operative report will serve as an important piece of legal evidence.

After I've dictated the operative report, Dr. Peterson and I walk out to the family waiting room. We are immediately descended upon by Mrs. Lazarra and Mrs. D'Annunzio's three daughters. Dr. Peterson and I stand shoulder-to shoulder as he answers all their questions.

"Yes," he assures them. "Everything went well."

CHAPTER 32

GENTLEMEN WITH ABDOMINAL PAIN

This week, we identify two patients in the Outpatient Clinic who would benefit from surgery: Mr. Israel Solomon and Mr. Avro Carter.

Mr. Solomon is a 50 year-old gentleman whom we saw in clinic, with a symptomatic right inguinal hernia. In the Operating Room Dr. Chung gives Mr. Solomon spinal anesthesia for the procedure. Chris Gable, Dr. Peterson and I scrub. Chris does the case and Dr. Peterson directs the operation. I am there to provide exposure, and to observe.

We enter the operating room and proceed with the operation. We identify the hernia, and Chris makes a sturdy repair with polypropylene mesh. The procedure proceeds smoothly with only a few milliliters of blood loss. Throughout the case I hear Peterson's relentless mantra directing Chris.

"Watch the tips of your dissecting scissors, watch what they're going to cut: use your left hand to pick up what you're going to sew, follow the curve of the needle; hold the tissues—don't crush them; be certain your knots go down square, do it the same way every time...."

This mantra may be one of the secrets of Peterson's technical prowess: do it carefully, and do it the same way every time. And bask in the partitas of Johan Sebastian Bach.

Forty minutes later we are finished, and we wheel Mr. Solomon's gurney into the Post Anesthesia Recovery Room. The spinal anesthesia and Valium are still exerting their magic; he's not yet moving his legs, and he's fast asleep.

"The operative report," I remind Chris. "Dictate it now, while it's fresh in your mind."

***

Our next case is Mr. Avro Carter, a rancher from the far west with a grapefruit-size mass on the back of his neck. He is accompanied by his wife. I find it hard to believe that anyone could ignore such a mass for four or five years, but the powers of denial are not to be underestimated.

"Where do they come from?" Mr. Carter asks. "Or perhaps I should ask—why do they develop?"

We have no idea, but the overwhelming majority of them are perfectly benign. Chris and I do the operation with Mr. Carter lying face down on the operating table. Peterson sits on a stool in the OR beside us, observing and offering advice. Mr. Carter is fully awake with a calming dose of Valium.

"We'll be working behind you," I tell Mr. Carter. "On the back of your neck. But we'll tell you everything we're going to do before we do it. No surprises: I promise."

That seems to relax him. After a brief warning, we inject the skin on the back of his neck with lidocaine, a local anesthetic. Chris uses a scalpel to make a transverse incision. Then I show him how to develop a plane of dissection between the grapefruit-size fatty mass and the muscles of the spine, and also stay out of some important nerves that run behind the neck. Occasionally we encounter a vein or artery that requires clamping, cutting and tying off with a suture, but most of the vessels are so small that they can be transected with the electrocautery. In just a few minutes we separate the fatty mass from the muscles, and we are able to hand it to the scrub nurse to be sent to the pathologist.

We now trim the skin flaps to fit properly against

the back of Mr. Carter's neck. We place a test tube-size suction drain to capture any oozing, and we wheel him into the PAR. After about an hour, we send Mr. Carter home after he promises to return at eight o'clock in the morning for us to remove the drain.

"Simple Surgery." Chris says triumphantly.

"Not so quick," I say. "Let's see how he does over the next couple of days. I remember how excited I felt after doing my first case, four years ago. Of course," I say, "Back in those days, the residents dictated the operative report immediately or else we used *Bulgarian anesthesia.*"

"*Bulgarian anesthesia?* What is *that?*"

"That's where we put a wooden bowl on your head and hit it with a hammer."

Chris laughs, but he gets the message.

***

The next morning I remove Mr. Carter's suction drain. It has been in place in the wound for about twelve hours. In spite of the brief duration, the wound drains thick, cloudy pus, the hall marks of a wound infection. How could it possibly become infected in such a short time? It may have been harboring the seeds of infection even before we operated.

Mr. Carter cannot reach around to the back of his neck, but his wife agrees to learn how to care for the wound. I give her a carton of four-by-four inch gauze pads, a box of dry sterile pads and a carton of rubber gloves. Then I show her how to pack the wound with wet-to-dry dressings, replacing the saline-moistened gauze pads every eight hours. We also culture the wound to determine what bacteria might be growing there, but that will require several days before we can identify the bacteria.

"We want the wound to heal from the inside-to-out, from the bottom-up", I explain. "We don't want to bottle up the infection; we want it to drain out. It's just going to take time, about six weeks.

"And when you take out the gauze pads," I tell his wife, "Mr. Carter can stand in the shower, and flush the

241

wound with soapy water. After he showers, you will be able to pack it for another eight hours. We will schedule you so we can see the wound on a regular basis, but you can call the Clinic any time you want us to see it between appointments. Our residents are in the hospital every day seven days a week, and you can also page me directly on any day."

I feel terrible about the wound infection, but we did everything we were supposed to do, when we were supposed to do it. We did not use preop antibiotics as he had no infections in the neck or elsewhere on his body, and no open wounds. If he had evidence of infection anywhere on his body, I would not have operated until the infection had resolved.

CHAPTER 33

POST-OP CLINIC

The first patient we see in follow-up clinic is Mrs. D'Annunzio. She is accompanied by her mother, the redoubtable Mrs. Lazarra, who arrives with a large shopping bag. Mrs. D'Annunzio's wound is clean and dry. She has no intra-abdominal symptoms. As they are about to leave, Mrs. Lazarra reaches into her shopping bag to present Dr. Peterson with a bottle of Lambrusco, a popular Italian red wine. Dr. Peterson is most gracious in accepting it, explaining that a gift is not necessary. But Mrs. Lazarra insists, and no one is willing to disagree with Mrs. Lazarra.

When we walk out of the examining room, Art looks at me with an annoyed expression. "We're the ones who should be getting the gift" he says. "We did the workup and sweated through that first night".

"Don't you worry," I tell him. "Our time will come."

We don't have long to wait, for, poised in the clinic waiting area, ready to pounce on us, is Mrs. Lazarra, insisting that we visit her at her *Italian Market* restaurant. We are to be her guests for dinner. How can I say no? Italians love to cook and I love to eat, especially really good Italian food.

"How thoughtful," I say, "But you really didn't have to..."

"You like Italian food?" she asks ignoring my protestations. Before I can answer, she says, "We have five veal dishes, six chicken dishes, ravioli, lasagna, eggplant, six kinds of homemade pasta, homemade biscotti and cannoli for dessert."

"But Mrs. Lazarra . . ."

"Next week," she says. "Come Tuesday, midweek, when we're not so busy. And bring the student doctors. You're all invited."

I thank her profusely. "Such a kind invitation. It isn't necessary, but we do appreciate it."

"Tut-tut," she says touching her index finger to her lips. "Seven o'clock, Tuesday."

Our second clinic patient is Mr. Solomon. Chris had repaired his right inguinal hernia. His wound looks clean and dry, and he has had no inflammation or undue postop discomfort. When we walk out of the examining room, Mr. Solomon turns to me.

"I appreciate what you fellows did for me," he says "and I have a little something for you in my car. How about walking out to the parking lot with me after clinic?"

"That's very nice of you, Mr. Solomon. But it's really not necessary. Besides, we won't be finished with clinic until after five o'clock."

"I'll wait," he insists. He takes a seat in the clinic waiting area, finds a stack of old National Inquirer magazines, and settles in to wait for us to finish seeing all our other patients. By the end of our clinic hours he'll be well versed in who in Hollywood has gained fifty pounds, and which actress is sleeping with whom.

***

Our last clinic patient is Mr. Avro Carter; the patient who had a giant lipoma on the back of his neck. He is accompanied by his wife. I tell them that we got the official report back from the pathologist, and it confirms our impression that the mass was just a benign fatty tumor—a lipoma. "I've never heard of one of these things becoming cancerous."

"Where do they come from?" Mr. Carter asks.

"We have no idea, but they are perfectly benign. If this one comes back or develops in a new location, you should be seen by a surgeon who can remove it."

"I will," he says. "I'll come see Dr. Peterson or yourself."

Mr. Carter turns to me and changes the subject. "Tell me doc, do you fish—*fly* fish, I mean? The real thing?"

"Can't say that I ever tried it."

"You really should give it a try. It can be very challenging."

"Yes, well, one of these days. . ."

"No, I mean you *really* should try it. I have some property in Idaho, on a branch of the Salmon River. I'm telling you, the streams are so chock full of trout; they're jumping out of the water. Even a beginner can't go wrong."

I must admit it's tempting. "How would we get there?" I ask.

"Well, we would fly into Salt Lake City, rent a car, and drive about three hundred miles north. Finally, we would ride in on horseback for a day to get to the streams. We'll camp out once we're there. I'll take care of everything." Mr. Carter grins as he anticipates an adventure with his doctor. I think most people would like to be social friends with their doctors.

A campsite on a branch of the Salmon River may be paradise for an outdoorsman like Mr. Carter, but riding a horse for eight hours going in, and another eight hours coming out sounds like pure agony for this city boy. I can see he's disappointed when I decline.

That reminds me, I've got to write myself a note to call Dr. Quinn's office. I need to list Mr. Carter's wound infection on next week's Morbidity and Mortality list. I hope Quinn is in a good mood these days. Maybe we'll be lucky and he will go on vacation.

***

After we've seen all the patients in clinic, and we are about to leave, I spy Mr. Solomon, still sitting patiently in the waiting area. I join him, and we walk out to the parking lot together.

"You may remember," he says. "I'm in the wholesale food business."

"Yes, I do remember."

"Do you like pickled herring?"

"Well, yes as a matter of fact, I do—as an appetizer, once in a while."

"Good," he says. "I brought you a case of pickled herring in sour cream sauce—12 jars. But you have to keep it refrigerated."

Twelve jars! What am I going to do with 12 refrigerated jars of pickled fish? I don't know 12 people who would eat more than one jar of the delicacy in their entire lifetime, and I certainly don't have a refrigerator at home large enough to hold 12 jars of pickled herring.

"I'd be delighted to have *one* jar," I say. "But really, that's all I can accept."

"Maybe you'd prefer herring in wine sauce," Mr. Solomon says, stepping back. "I have a case of it, just for you." He points to a second case of 12 jars in his trunk.

"Please," I say. "I appreciate your offer, but I must decline. One jar is more than enough." Privately, I hope Mr. Solomon never develops another hernia; who knows what exotic food that would bring.

***

One week later, after evening rounds, I gather our team of residents and students, and we drive out to Mrs. Lazarra's *Italian Market* restaurant. Dr. Peterson also was invited, but he says he has other matters to attend to. In the restaurant, we are greeted by Mrs. Lazarra and Mrs. D'Annunzio. Mrs. Lazarra comments that we look different without our white lab coats, but I assure her that it is us, her friends from the hospital. Everyone laughs a little, uncertain as to what is proper etiquette in circumstances such as these.

Mrs. Lazarra provides everyone with a glass of Chianti and a menu. She asks if we have any special requests for dinner—veal, pasta, red sauce, sausage, whatever we wish. We tell her, but neither she nor her staff records anything we say. After about 20 minutes, a contingent of dark-haired Italian waiters arrives to deliver our food, one mammoth dinner plate after another of virtually every entrée listed on the menu.

"Mrs. Lazarra," I protest. "What are we going to do with all this food?"

"You'll eat what you can, and what you can't, you'll take home—*mangia, mangia...eat, eat.*"

"This is so kind of you."

"And it was kind of you when you came in during the middle of the night to see my daughter."

I am about to say that it is my responsibility, that we are *supposed* to come in to see sick patients. That's certainly the truth but, of course, none of us is willing to argue with a determined Mrs. Lazarra.

PHILIP B. DOBRIN, M.D.

CHAPTER 34

APPENDICITIS

I am standing in the Emergency Room with Chris Gabel, Art Mortiz, Veronica and Gary, the last two being medical students assigned to our service. We have been called to see Mr. Nichols, a twenty-two year old man who came to the Emergency Room with complaints of abdominal pain.

Veronica interviewed him while I was in the Institutional Review Board (IRB) meeting, and she presents him to us now. "He was awakened early this morning by vague pain located near his belly button."

"His *belly button*? You can do better than that, Veronica. Dr. Peterson will be here any minute. He'll eat you alive for calling it a belly button. Speak like a doctor. It's an *umbilicus*."

"All right," she says impatiently. "An umbilicus."

I can see she isn't taking me seriously, but Peterson will be here any minute. She won't be able to say I didn't warn her. "What did Mr. Nichols have for dinner?" I ask.

"I'm not sure...no, wait. He didn't have dinner. That's it. He wasn't hungry."

What's the significance of that?" I ask.

"I'm not sure," she says.

"What diagnoses are we considering here?"

Veronica thinks, her eyes searching.

"Bowel obstruction?"

"Could be, especially if he's had abdominal surgery in the past. Has he had abdominal surgery?"

She thinks for a moment. "I'm trying to remember if I saw a scar on his abdomen." She struggles through her memory. "No. No scar."

"So is it likely that he has a bowel obstruction?"

"Could be, but probably not."

I give her a little help. "How about an internal hernia that's become trapped or twisted."

"Oh, yes. Okay," she says.

"That could cause a bowel obstruction even without a past external hernia, but it's kind of rare."

"What other diagnoses should we be considering in this patient?"

"Diverticulosis and diverticulitis?'

"Is he the usual age for a patient who develops diverticulosis?"

"I don't think so. He's too young."

"Right. Now, what else should we consider? Think about a high probability diagnosis."

Veronica puts on an inquiring expression. "Inflammatory bowel disease?"

She's asking me to answer questions instead of the other way around. This is like pulling teeth. "How about if I give you a clue?"

Veronica nods.

"Okay, then how about pain elicited in the left lower quadrant when you put gentle pressure on the right side?"

"That suggests peritonitis, inflammation of the peritoneum on the right side," she says. "Right?"

"Right. And a likely cause of it in a man of this age?"

"Appendicitis."

At last. "Good for you. You know what they say: when you're searching for a diagnosis look for horses, not zebras."

Veronica is smiling. I guess she likes horses.

Dr. Peterson shows up, and listens carefully to Veronica as she recites the patient's medical history. He doesn't even flinch when she uses the words *belly button*. I'll have to speak to him about that.

She's not done yet.

Veronica nods. "There is so much to remember."

"How about his blood work?" I ask her.

"His white count is up–twelve thousand"

"What would you think if I told you it was twenty thousand per milliliter? Would that make you worry?"

"I'm not sure," she says.

"Well, if it were my white count, I would worry. And what I'd worry about is a *perforated* appendicitis, leaking pus or stool into the abdomen.

"Sounds like trouble," Veronica says.

"You bet it is."

"How about x-rays?" Peterson asks. "Do x-rays give you a lot of help in making a diagnosis of appendicitis?"

"Plain films don't" Chris says. "But a carefully done barium enema can help. If the infused barium flows all the way out to the tip of the appendix that pretty much rules out appendicitis, but even that is not one hundred percent accurate. Appendicitis really is a *clinical* diagnosis.

"But sometimes you can spot a fecalith," he says. "That's a small hardened mass of stool that blocks the lumen of the appendix, so that the appendix can't empty. Some people think that that is the cause of appendicitis."

Everybody does a little shuffle, tired of standing and speculating as to what Mr. Nichol's problem might be.

"Let's go see the patient," Peterson says.

We all troop into the examining room where Chris introduces us to Mr. Nichols.

When we lay our hands on Mr. Nichols' abdomen, there is no doubt that he has peritonitis, sensitive to even the lightest external touch, the slightest motion or cough. He also has marked rebound tenderness. I suspect appendicitis, but a disconcerting finding is that the maximum sensitivity is in the *left* quadrant, not the right, the usual location of the appendix.

Next, we perform a rectal examination, and we find the same thing—maximum sensitivity is in Mr. Nichol's left lower quadrant, not his right. This could be an indicator of pathology that does not involve the appendix. Perhaps he has inflammatory bowel disease, a well-known young person's ailment. In any case, Mr. Nichols has an acutely tender abdomen that requires surgical exploration. We talk it over with him, and he accepts a high likelihood of appendicitis or inflammatory bowel disease. He also accepts the need for exploration of the abdomen. I alert the operating room and the anesthesiology department to get things ready. Then I mobilize the service to get the consent forms signed, and the history and physical examinations completed. After we push and pull what seems like every stubborn step, we finally get Mr. Nichols into the operating room.

We stand at the sink outside the operating room, scrubbing for surgery. Our medical students scrub beside us, eager to see the operation, and Dr. Peterson uses the opportunity to review some important points with the students. "The appendix is a cylinder of intestine that extends like a pencil out of the right intestine. It can point in any direction, and it may be covered by peritoneum. Appendicitis entails inflammation of that pencil-like projection.

"A diagnosis of appendicitis is one of the most common reasons we explore a patient's abdomen. The periumbilical pain often is accompanied by nausea, vomiting and loss of appetite. We're not certain why the loss of appetite, but it seems to be a common finding. Over the course of several hours, the pain usually migrates from the umbilicus to the right lower quadrant. This migration away from the periumbilical area is characteristic of acute appendicitis, but migration of discomfort to the left lower quadrant is unusual, and suggests an entirely different etiology for the pain—perhaps inflammatory bowel disease like Crohn's disease, a difficult inflammatory disease of the bowel."

After we scrub, we enter the operating room, scrub and drape Mr. Nichol's abdomen, and gather around the operating table. We make a horizontal abdominal incision.

"In a child or a teenager," Peterson says, "We would make a diagonal incision so small that it could be covered by a bikini bottom. But in an older patient or in any patient where the diagnosis is uncertain, we usually use a transverse incision to give us more room to maneuver, if we need to."

Now we go to work. Once we have entered the abdomen, we examine the intra-abdominal organs. Except for the cecum at the base of the right colon, the intra-abdominal organs appear normal. There is evidence of inflammation at the base of the cecum, the origin of the appendix. We dissect and mobilize the right intestine. In so doing, we find an inflamed, but intact, appendix that does not appear to have perforated or leaked into the abdominal cavity. Mr. Nichols is in luck. Also, he has an unusually long appendix, part of which is concealed behind the cecum. After we free it from the surrounding connective tissue, we find that the appendix reaches from the right side (which is normal and expected) to extend all the way across the abdomen to reach the left side. That explains why Mr. Nichols' tenderness observed during the abdominal and rectal examinations was located on Mr. Nichols's left side. We excise the inflamed pencil-like appendix and oversew the cecum to enclose the appendiceal stump. We thoroughly irrigate the abdomen to dilute and cleanse it of bacteria. Finally, we close the abdomen with strong, slowly-absorbable stitches

We send the excised appendix to the pathologist for his evaluation. In spite of much speculation, no one really knows the normal physiological purpose of the appendix.

Peterson turns to Chris and says, "Suppose we operated and found a normal appendix. What would you do then? Would you excise the appendix, or leave it alone?"

Chris contemplates the question for a few seconds,

and then says that he would remove the suspicious organ. "If anyone saw that scar on his right lower quadrant, they would assume that his appendix had been removed."

"That's the right answer." Peterson says. He goes on to explain, "Because the clues to the diagnosis are so often subtle, a false-positive rate of 10-12 percent is desirable to avoid missing appendicitis. In other words, we would rather over-diagnose appendicitis in a normal appendix, rather than fail to diagnose it in an inflamed appendix."

I remind Chris to dictate the operative report, write post-op orders and we hurry off to an early lunch. Oh, if only every day went this well. As we are leaving the operating room area, I watch as Peterson leans over to make a quiet comment. "Veronica," he says. "The word is *umbilicus,* not *belly button"*

***

At a few minutes before one, we head out to Dr. Peterson's afternoon clinic.

"This is how it works," I explain to the students. "We usually have twenty-five or thirty scheduled patients, plus a few add-ons. We see each patient before Peterson does. We get their medical history, examine them and make a tentative diagnosis. Then we present the patient to Dr. Peterson."

Wait a moment. Wasn't it just a month or so ago that Barney and Nathan outlined this same routine to me? No, it was *five years* ago! How the years have flitted by.

"Now," I say to Veronica and Gary. "Listen to the patient's medical history. That's where we get most of our diagnostic clues. Some patients think that the more symptoms they can pile on, the more seriously we will take them. They don't realize that we correlate a diversity of signs and symptoms with specific clinical diseases. It's a cognitive jigsaw puzzle that we try to solve without being able to see the pieces laid out flat on the dining room table."

CHAPTER 35

BOWEL OBSTRUCTION

We sit in the second floor nurses' station waiting for Dr. Peterson to call with his usual list of morning problems. Today, he directs us to go to the surgical floor to see Mr. Pappas, a new admission.

George Pappas is an energetic 60-year old Greek businessman, the executive of his own company. He is in the hospital for abdominal pain, but you might never know it when we you meet him as he is hard at work. His hospital bed is covered with shipping documents and business forms, and he has taken over the unoccupied hospital bed next to him for use as a work table.

Mr. Pappas has a past 6-year medical history of abdominal surgery for colon cancer. He complains of abdominal distention, some moderate pain and difficulty in passing gas or stool. Taken together, his history and symptoms suggest obstruction of the small bowel.

Mr. Pappas speaks just a few words of English, but he is accompanied by his English-speaking daughters, Anna and Sophia Pappas. According to his daughters, Mr. Pappas had surgery six years ago in Greece. The surgery was a success and proceeded without complications, but a few weeks after the procedure Mr. Pappas developed a postoperative small bowel obstruction or *paralytic ileus,* as it is sometimes called in medical parlance. Sophia tells us that after about a week in the hospital in Greece, vigorous arguments developed between Mr. Pappas and his doctors. His surgeons wanted to take him back to the operating room to relieve the obstruction, but Mr. Pappas refused. In the end, his symptoms of obstruction resolved without surgical intervention. But, the differences between Mr. Pappas and his doctors persisted and became so intense that eventually, he and his doctors were no longer on speaking terms.

Since that time Mr. Pappas has been without symptoms. However, in the last few days he has again become distended with symptoms suggestive of an acute small bowel obstruction. X-rays currently taken at University Hospital are consistent with that diagnosis. His permanent long term medical records remain in Greece.

Physical examination demonstrates that Mr. Pappas's abdomen is distended and somewhat tender to palpation. Listening to his abdomen with a stethoscope reveals high-pitched bowel sounds, an indication that the bowel is actively contracting, attempting to propel intestinal contents through the bowel. Mr. Pappas has a slight fever and a minimal elevation of white blood cell count, both signs of mild inflammation. X-ray pictures of his abdomen show distended loops of bowel with air/fluid levels, i.e. a layer of fluid and above that, a layer of air. This multilayered appearance is a classic x-ray sign of small bowel obstruction.

After we examine Mr. Pappas, we explain that we plan to treat him conservatively with IV fluids, intravenous hyperalimentation, and nasogastric decompression with a naso-gastric tube in his nose and stomach. We explain that most of the air seen in the small bowel on x-ray actually is air he swallowed; much of it is removed by using a naso-gastric tube connected to suction. In return, Mr. Pappas makes a long, impassioned speech through Anna and Sophia explaining that under no circumstances will he consent to undergo additional surgery. He insists that it is unnecessary, and that all he requires is some pain medication and sufficient time to *heal.* We refuse to provide him with pain medication to avoid camouflaging his symptoms. But it becomes abundantly clear that Mr. Pappas is fiercely independent.

We insert a naso-gastric tube, and place it on intermittent suction. We also explain that bowel obstructions frequently are caused by bands of scar tissue that develop during or after the healing process; these bands can become wrapped around the normal intestine cutting off its blood supply. If these do not release spontaneously they must be removed surgically. Finally, we explain that surgery for bowel obstruction often requires nothing more than a judicious snip of one or two exuberant bands of scar. But Mr. Pappas ignores what we say. He doggedly refuses surgery, and poses a penetrating question.

"What will prevent new scar tissue from forming to again bind the bowel?" he asks? "It has happened before."

"Many patients develop an obstruction just once or twice." Dr. Peterson answers. "Other patients are prone to repeated episodes of bowel obstruction. But in any case, trapped segments of bowel cannot just be ignored without risking permanent loss of several inches of the bowel."

Dr. Peterson and I discuss Mr. Pappas' situation, and we agree that, with his tendency to form postoperative obstructions, it would be wise to give him a trial of conservative therapy, but we also agree that if a relentless bowel obstruction does not resolve, we should operate promptly to relieve it.

Dr. Peterson encourages me to be patient. "He is a smart man," Peterson says. "And there is not much we can do if he refuses surgery. But, you mark my words; he will change his mind if he develops increased abdominal pain."

Dr. Peterson is smart and experienced, and I greatly respect his judgment, but in this case, I'm not sure he's got it right. Mr. Pappas seems to have made up his mind, and in his culture and in his business, he is the boss.

Over the next several days, Mr. Pappas's abdominal tenderness increases. At the same time, his body temperature and his white blood cell count begin to rise. These are the signs of increasing inflammation and likely intra-abdominal inflammation.

We ask for a family meeting to discuss his medical condition. At that meeting, Dr. Peterson reiterates that a loop of bowel may become trapped and require no more than a few small snips to release the scar tissue, or it may require resection of an entire loop of bowel. It all depends on what is found at surgery. But without intra-abdominal exploration we cannot know just what is required. Anna and Sophia understand the reasons for our request, and they reluctantly agree to discuss it with their father. Mr. Pappas stares blankly at us during the conference. I don't know why, but I suspect that as a long-standing negotiator in the business world, he understands much of what is being said, even when we speak English.

"It's been five years since he had an operation," Sophia says. "Isn't it unusual to have this problem so long after surgery?"

"That often is true," I tell her. "Many bowel obstructions occur soon after surgery, but others may occur much later. Just recently, we had a lady with a loop of bowel caught in scar tissue that did not occur until 18 years after surgery."

Anna and Sophia meet with their father in his hospital room for a family conference while the rest of us withdraw from their discussion. The door to his room closes with a resounding click. But the meeting is calamitous, and the ensuing arguments can be heard throughout the surgical floor. I can identify Anna and Sophia's voices by their loudness and their tone of desperation. I really don't have much hope when the daughters emerge tearfully from their conference. Their father will not alter his position; he is convinced that he will recover spontaneously, as he did after the original surgery in Greece.

"He is so stubborn," Anna says tearfully. "He won't listen to anybody."

Over the next two days, Mr. Pappas does not improve. Instead, he becomes feverish with a rapid pulse, and his blood exhibits increasing acidosis, a critical sign of dying bowel. Moreover, the high-pitched bowel sounds heard in his abdomen earlier have become weak and less frequent.

"You must convince him," I tell the daughters. "If he continues on his present path, I'm afraid he will not survive."

Dr. Peterson offers a sober assessment when he says, "Your father is practicing medicine without having gone to medical school; he is acting as both the patient and his own doctor."

"This is all we can do," Sophia says.

***

This morning we arrive at the hospital to find Mr. Pappas unconscious and unresponsive. His daughters find themselves bound in conflict. In light of his often-repeated wishes, they disagree as to what medically should be done.

"He is very firm as to what he wants," Anna says. "He does not want to have surgery."

"But that is the only way he will survive," Sophia says.

"How will he feel?" Anna asks. "When he wakes up and realizes that he had surgery, in spite of his wishes?"

"He will be alive," Sophia answers sharply.

"We made what we thought was the best decision we could."

Sophia asks a more disquieting question. "What if we don't give the doctors permission to do surgery, and he dies?"

The two daughters struggle briefly in silence. Finally, they reluctantly fill out the necessary paperwork giving Dr. Peterson permission to perform exploratory surgery.

"In the old days," he says, "when we encountered

this kind of situation patients' *next of kin* were able to grant permission to the doctors to perform whatever life-saving treatments were required.

"More recently, *next of kin* designation has been replaced by a more specific *Power of Attorney for Health Care*, a document that gives medical decision-making powers to his designate if a patient becomes incapable of making medical decisions for himself."

***

It is a hurried trip we take to the operating room.

We open Mr. Pappas's abdomen from just below the sternum to just above the bladder. This provides us with excellent access to the abdominal cavity. But the moment we open the fascia we immediately are assaulted by the nauseating stench of dying tissue—a loop of small bowel has been trapped by tough fibrous bands impeding the blood supply. We clamp above and below the compromised loop and excise the dying tissue.

Then we systematically inspect every inch of small and large bowel that we can reach by passing the loops of intestine hand over hand, snipping bands of scar wherever they appear to be restricting the intestine. Some of these are as tough as violin strings. We leave innocent bands alone, concerned that they will heal by forming new restrictive bands.

We then restore intestinal continuity by sewing the cut small bowel end-to-end. We take multiple cultures of the abdominal cavity. Then we wash out the abdomen with 40 liters of warm sterile saline.

Next, we close the fascia, the deep layers of the abdominal wall. This pulls the tough fascia together at the base of the wound, and keeps the bowel in the abdomen. We pack that area superficial to the fascia with clean gauze as we did on Avro Carter, renewing those dressings three times each day to decrease the risk of developing a wound infection.

It is hard to believe that such an unimpressive band of scar could produce so much injury. We close Mr. Pappas's abdomen with double stranded stainless steel wire, a suture that is strong and resistant to infection.

Immediately after surgery we discuss all aspects of the situation with Anna and Sofia Pappas. Their response is hopeful, but realistic. Now, they both are convinced they made the right decision to explore their father's abdomen. We transfer Mr. Pappas to the Surgical Intensive Care Unit. There, he teeters on the edge of life. Mr. Pappas's respiration is supported by a ventilator, his nutrition is supported intravenously by hyperalimentation, and the infection in his abdomen and his blood is battled by IV fluids and antibiotics. These treatments may support his life, but they may not be capable of restoring his *health*.

After we leave the family, Peterson offers his opinion to the students.

"For each organ system that fails there is a 25 to 30 percent increase in mortality. But don't be fooled. Mr. Pappas is a tough old bird, and he is used to winning. My bet is that he'll make it."

PHILIP B. DOBRIN, M.D.

CHAPTER 36

PERFORATED DUODENAL ULCER

I'm on the phone speaking with Chris Gabel, telling him about our attending coverage situation.

"Dr. Peterson is attending a conference downtown," I tell him. "And he won't be available except for life-threatening emergencies. So let's stay out of trouble; we're going to be on our own."

Stay out of trouble. The only way for Chris to stay out of trouble is to not be here. If he roams around the hospital he's bound to find something that needs attention.

Just as soon as I hang up the phone, Chris calls me right back with a problem. "I'm in the Burn Unit", he says. "Seeing a patient named William Sayer. Do you know him?"

"No."

"He was admitted to the Burn Unit with a 20 percent burn to his hands, face and chest; he had a back-yard trash fire that got away from him. He's been an inpatient for about a week, and he's been doing very well. But today, without warning, he developed signs of an acute abdomen with exquisite tenderness and board-like rigidity."

I call our medical students, Veronica and Gary, and we head to the Burn Unit. There we meet Tom Mount

Royal, the junior resident currently assigned to the burn unit. He greets us and introduces us to Mr. Sayer.

Upon physical examination, we find Mr. Sayer exactly as Chris described him, complete with exquisite abdominal tenderness to palpation. Reaching forward to gently grasp Mr. Sayer's hips, and then gently rocking him to and fro elicits an impressive indication of abdominal tenderness. According to Tom, these signs have been present only for the last hour or so.

I ask the students to examine Mr. Sayer, but *be gentle*, I insist. "I have a question for Chris and the students. When we came into the Unit we passed six or seven patients with a variety of burns. Did any of you notice any differences between Mr. Sayer and the other patients?"

The medical students stare at each other with a puzzled look. "All right," I say to Tom, "You tell us; has Mr. Sayer received any treatments that are different from what your burn patients usually receive?"

"Yes," he says. "Mr. Sayer was treated according to our usual Burn treatment protocol, but with one exception; he refused to let us put a naso-gastric tube through his nose and into his stomach and duodenum. We explained to him that using a naso-gastric tube is a good way to provide continuous nutrition, and to prevent the development of a gastroduodenal ulcer. I remember Dr. Wisniewski telling us that, in the days before the Burn Unit used naso-gastric tubes, several of the patients developed stress ulcers. But since the Burn Unit has been using naso-gastric tubes, they haven't had a single GI bleed or perforation. Whether this was due to the nutrition provided or dilution of the acid in gastroduodenal environment is unclear. We tried to convince him to use the tube but he absolutely refused. He insisted it would be too uncomfortable.

"We tried to talk him into it, pointed out the therapeutic advantages of the tube, but he still refused. He insisted that he has never had an ulcer, and that he has never been treated for an ulcer."

We stand for a moment in thoughtful silence, each person mulling over the situation. We all try to do the right thing for our patients, but if a patient refuses our recommendations, then we really cannot do too much about it.

"How about some x-rays of the abdomen," I ask Tom.

"Coming right up," he says. "I'll bet you've never seen anything like this."

And he is quite right, for just beneath the left and right diaphragms, are two baseball-size collections of free air, air that is in the abdomen but outside the small or large bowel, somewhere it does not belong. With Mr. Sayer's medical history, I am guessing that that there has been a perforation of the duodenum.

I explain matters to the students. If a patient has a duodenal ulcer, and it erodes *posteriorly* it is likely to injure the pancreaticoduodenal artery. Patients with this problem often have bleeding of bright red blood. In fact, it can be life-threatening hemorrhage. On the other hand, duodenal ulcers that erode *anteriorly* result in a perforation of the duodenal wall. This spills the duodenal contents into the free peritoneal space. Hence the free air and the acute abdomen, but without a great deal of bleeding. Whatever the cause, a patient displaying such severe peritoneal signs deserves an exploratory laparotomy, and the sooner the better.

The students listen intently, acknowledging my explanation.

It is time to page Dr. Peterson, to type and cross match blood in case it is needed, inform anesthesia that we need to go to the OR and ask them to see Mr. Sayer, and get the surgical and blood consents signed. Time is critical because spilling bowel contents outside of the gastrointestinal tract will contaminate the entire abdominal cavity with acid, bacteria and digestive secretions; this will produce life-threatening peritonitis.

***

I am standing in the Burn Unit nurses' station, phone in hand, waiting for someone in the OR suite to pick up my call.

There! At last someone picks it up. Rats. It's my nemesis, LeRay. She is the clerk at the desk tonight. A cooperative word from her is as rare as rocking horse manure. She sounds bored; she *always* sounds bored. Or maybe it's lack of interest.

"What is the operation?" she asks.

"Exploratory laparotomy."

"Who should I list as the attending?"

"Peterson,"

"It can't be. Peterson's out of town."

"Yes, well, he's *supposed* to be out of town, but he's still here, and he said he'd come in for emergencies like this."

"Well, that's nice of him. But I can't give you permission to operate with an attending who isn't here, and has no intention of being here."

"Oh, he'll be here."

"Well, I'll have to see him to believe it."

"LeRay, this patient, Mr. Sayer, is leaking intestinal contents into his abdomen. People *die* from that. We need to do a laparotomy, get in there and control the leak."

"All right," she says with a sigh. "How do you spell laparotomy?"

"Just like it sounds, l-a-p-a-r-o-t... oh, never mind." Let's just go, I think to myself as I shift my weight from one foot to the other.

"All right, but first I have to fill out the form."

"What form is that?"

"You know, the new emergency surgery form."

"What's that all about?"

"Don't blame me. It's Surgery's form, not ours."

It is silent on the phone. I can hear LeRay's breathing followed by her usual bored yawn as she hangs up the receiver. Life for her must be oh-so-boring. I call her back.

"It's me again. Now don't hang up on me."

"What do you mean don't hang up on you? You hung up on me."

"Whatever you say. I just want to get started."

Just then my pager goes off. At last, Peterson.

I tell him what we have observed clinically and my impressions. I keep LeRay's tank-trap personality to myself. Peterson agrees with my impressions and wishes me good luck.

"Now for the bad news," he says. There's no way that I'm going to be able to get out of this meeting tonight. You'll have to rely on a back-up attending to cover you. I really can't just show up, present my talk and walk out. I'll call Mary-Beth Kennedy and let her know. She is the attending covering the OR for emergencies tonight. Have you ever scrubbed with her?"

"No, I never have."

"Oh. You'll like her. She is very patient. She will scrub with you but she will turn the case over to you. You'll see. I'll drop by when I get finished with our meeting to see how you're doing."

***

What I first notice about Dr. Kennedy is her slight stature. She is just over five feet. In fact, in order to reach Mr. Sayers she will have to stand on a stack of platforms placed beside the operating table. What I notice next is her profound, crippling limp. I've heard that it is due to polio contracted when she was a child—what a courageous soul.

***

"Well," I ask LeRay. "When are we going to get started?"

"Stop pestering me. You'll start as soon as they finish the case they are doing in there now."

"And just when might that be?"

267

"I'd guess in about half an hour, just as soon as Dr. Goldstein finishes his appendectomy."

"Dr. Goldstein!" One way or another, it's always Lenny.

***

I use the delay to make a phone call to Mr. Sayer's family explaining the situation. They appreciate my call and tell me that they will come to the hospital as soon as they can

After a 45 minute delay we finally are in the operating room. Mr. Sayer is lying on the operating table receiving a dose of antibiotics.

Right now, Chris is scrubbing Mr. Sayer's abdomen while Dr. Hakeem begins his anesthesia routine. Dr. Kennedy and I are gowned and gloved waiting for Chris to finish. When he does, we drape Mr. Sayer, and I make a midline abdominal incision from his rib cage down to just above his bladder. We open the abdomen and perform a rapid-fire survey of the intra-abdominal organs.

Dr. Kennedy is a wonderful first assistant, guiding me but not taking over the case. As we progress we identify an opening in the duodenum, partially covered by a portion of the omentum, the fatty apron-like structure that hangs from the stomach.

For reasons that I cannot explain, the omentum is attracted to defects in the bowel wall. I use scissors to free up that attachment, then carefully place interrupted silk stitches to secure a fresh segment of omentum to cover the defect.

"So what do you want to do now?" Dr. Kennedy asks. "Do you want to do a definitive ulcer operation?"

"I've been thinking about it," I answer. "But Sayer has no history of ulcer disease, and I'd rather not do an anastomsis in an contaminated field." And I can't help but remember the surgical truism that *a satisfactory operation in a live patient is better than a perfect operation in a dead man.*"

We wash out the contaminated abdomen with 20 liters of warm sterile saline. Then I ask Chris to come to my side of the table, and close the irrigated abdomen. We use double-stranded stainless steel wire sutures, generally thought to be resistant to infection.

Chris seems to savor this operation, and, in a way, this has been his case from its discovery forward. As he labors, I can hear my voice echo Dr. Peterson's mantra; *Be certain you can see what you're sewing. Hold the forceps with your left hand. Rotate your wrist to follow the curvature of the needle...*

PHILIP B. DOBRIN, M.D.

CHAPTER 37

GRAND ROUNDS

It is ten minutes to eight on a Saturday morning, Lenny and I have finished morning rounds, and we are headed to the university amphitheater. We are going to Surgical Grand Rounds. Every Saturday morning a member of the Department of Surgery, or an invited guest, presents Grand Rounds, a one hour review of a topic of interest to surgeons.

"I'm scheduled to give Grand Rounds in two weeks," I tell Lenny. "But I don't have the slightest idea what to talk about."

"You've got two weeks? Then it's a piece of cake."

For Lenny everything's *a piece of cake.*

"Just take one of your current cases," he says. "Describe the patient, show some x-rays, throw in a few pearls of surgical wisdom, and you've got it made."

"Maybe," I muse. "But I can't just get up there and talk about hernias and hemorrhoids. I have to be *revealing, enlightening, inspiring,* not cause irreversible narcolepsy."

"Something will turn up," Lenny says. "You'll see. It always does." We arrive at the amphitheater, and now we have to decide where to sit, preferably where we'll be out of the limelight. Lenny and I find two seats in the last row, in the back of the amphitheater. A young male medical student sits down beside us.

This morning's speaker is Dr. Adolph Blum, Professor of Plastic Surgery. He's a visiting professor from another university, and his talk is a tiptoe down Ego-Trip Lane, an hour-long presentation of slides showing cosmetic surgery of ungainly noses and aging eyes before and after Blum has applied his reconstructive magic. It's all very aesthetic, but after thirty minutes of looking at before and after pictures of his handiwork, I'm gradually becoming anesthetized. Dr. Blum has the uncanny ability to squeeze five seconds of new ideas in 60 boring minutes. He's drowning us with examples, examples, examples, and I feel my eyelids closing, closing, and closing. So far, I'm following his presentation, but when Blum asks the projectionist to put on his *second* carousel of 80 additional slides, I'm overcome by a wave of desperation. How will I stay awake?

I turn and whisper to Lenny, "This is a new diagnosis—*Death by Toxic Lecture.* I'm going to the men's room. When Blum is finished, come out and cut me down."

"Oh, no you don't," Lenny says. "If you leave, I'm going with you."

"Shhh..." the medical student sitting next to us says. He turns and glares in our direction.

"Mind your own business," I tell him. "The stuff Blum is talking about is a review of his own work. It's not going to be on your exam."

"It's not? Well, in that case..." The medical student stands up and walks out.

"Now you've done it," Lenny says. "All three of us can't walk out at the same time. Blum might be offended, and whoever it was on our faculty who invited him will kill us. It might even have been Dr. Quinn."

"Dr. Quinn! The Grand Inquisitor of M and M? We certainly don't want to get him angry with us." I can just imagine a riled up Quinn at his M and M conference. He would be a regular Torquemada himself. No, we'd better just sit here and wait it out.

After another soporific half hour, Blum concludes his talk. There's a polite ripple of applause as the residents and the attending surgeons sitting in the front rows ask a few questions to demonstrate their interest.

"What's the incidence of infection?" someone asks.

"What's the recurrence rate?" Someone else asks.

"How do you treat infections?" A junior resident asks.

Dr. Blum is highly experienced, and he handles these questions like the professional that he is. But when I'm up there giving *my* presentation, I don't expect everyone to be so civilized. I'm one of their residents, and it will be *open season* with me as the target.

When Grand Rounds are over and the group disperses, I retreat to the medical school library. There, I bury myself behind a mountain of books and journals, and start scanning the tables of contents for something new and unusual I can talk about.

At three o'clock, Chris Gabel, the first year resident on our service, calls to tell me about a patient who has come into the ER. I can imagine Chris's milk bottle-thick glasses bobbing up and down on his little snub nose as he talks. "You've got to see this guy, Mr. Gulliver," Chris says. "He has fever and chills, and a foreign body in his flank. Looks like a surgical sponge on x-ray."

I walk over to the Emergency Room where I meet Mr. Gulliver, a taciturn, seventy year-old man with intense back pain. His eyes are glazed and vaguely focused. His face is flushed and feverish. He has shaking chills, a sign of sepsis, and lab tests that suggest that he may have bacteria in his blood. His white blood count is about twice normal. Somewhere in this man there is serious infection.

"Mr. Gulliver is from New York," Chris tells me. "Came out to visit family, and while he was here, broke a tooth at the gum line and needed oral surgery. That's about it."

"Past medical history?"

"A lumbar sympathectomy done 40 years ago for vascular disease in the legs. I've never heard much about that procedure."

"You wouldn't. Nobody does it for vascular insufficiency anymore. It interrupts the nerves that cause vessels in the skin to constrict, but it doesn't increase blood flow to the muscle the way everyone thought it would."

I carefully examine Mr. Gulliver. His physical examination is normal except for a long, well-healed scar on his flank, the site of the previously performed lumbar sympathectomy.

Then Chris shows me the results of a urinalysis that he ordered to rule out a urinary tract infection, and a chest x-ray that he ordered to rule out pneumonia. There is no evidence of infection at either site, but the film does reveal a foreign body, a four-by-four inch surgical sponge in the abdomen, near the kidney. It's just about where someone would make an incision to perform a lumbar sympathectomy. The sponge seems to be located directly beneath the surgical scar, but somewhat deeper.

"Let's get some x-rays of the flank," I tell Chris. "But tape a couple of coins on the scar to help us localize the sponge."

We send Mr. Gulliver back to X-ray for more films. While we're waiting, Chris and I talk, and I take advantage of the teaching opportunity. "Why do you think it got infected now, after all these years?" I ask him.

"The dental work?"

"Probably. When disturbed by the dental procedure, bacteria in the mouth enter the blood stream and stick to foreign bodies like the sponge. I've heard it said that the mouth is the second most unclean opening in the body."

"The guy who did his surgery did so forty years ago," Chris says. "I don't know how anybody could be so dumb as to leave a sponge in. Must be a moron."

"Well, nobody intends to leave a sponge in the wound, and we do everything we can to avoid it, but a blood-soaked sponge in the abdomen looks remarkably like dissected tissue. The sponge just seems to 'disappear'."

"Well, how about the instrument and sponge count the OR nurses do before we close? Don't they do that to be sure that we haven't left anything?"

"Yes, but it's pretty hectic when you're closing, and occasionally the nurses miscount. That's why they count and recount several times. An erroneous *correct* count gives us a false sense of security that everything is okay. In fact, what do you think the nurse's sponge and instrument count is in virtually every case of a retained object?"

Chris pushes his glasses up on his nose, and thinks for a moment. "The count is correct?"

"Exactly. Otherwise we'd keep on looking for whatever is missing. We'd even get a portable x-ray film to locate it."

When we get the x-rays back, we can see that the retained sponge is deep, but fortunately, it's located directly beneath the old scar. We start Mr. Gulliver on intravenous antibiotics; I show him the x-ray and explain the need to remove the sponge.

"He stares at me wide-eyed. How could it be there all these years and only now is a problem?"

I explain to him that the bacteria probably entered his blood stream during the dental work and stuck to the sponge.

"But forty years," he says. "That must be a new record."

"I think it must be," I say, and he seems proud to know that his foreign body set a "new land speed record." It always amazes me how patients seem to take satisfaction in knowing that they have the *first* or the *largest* or the *worst* whatever it is they have.

"The doctor said it was the worst case he'd ever seen." Nobody wants to have just a routine illness.

Mr. Gulliver is not eager to undergo surgery, but he realizes the necessity of removing the foreign body. We obtain his surgical consent, discuss his case with our attending, Dr. Peterson, on the telephone, and take Mr. Gulliver to the operating room

After he has been anesthetized and his airway has been secured, we turn him over onto his stomach, and then make an incision directly through the old scar.

Chris does the case with my assistance while Dr. Peterson stands nearby and watches us operate. He peppers us with questions and advice and the Peterson mantra. It should be a simple case if we can avoid excessive bleeding. Controlling bleeding in the depths of a deep hole can be difficult, and I urge Chris to stay in the middle of the scar as he dissects deeper and deeper. After a few minutes, we come upon the four-by-four sponge sitting in a pool of creamy white pus. After removing the sponge, we take cultures to send to the microbiology lab, and irrigate the wound with twenty liters of sterile saline until it appears to be clean. The wound is a deep crevasse, so we place a suction drain in it to its depths. Then we pack the wound down to its deepest point with fresh gauze which we count, and leave the wound open. We cover it with sterile bandages and ask the anesthesiologist to reverse the anesthesia.

Mr. Gulliver will be on his stomach or standing up for the next several weeks, and we will observe his wound and follow his laboratory data. The plan for postoperative care of the wound is straight forward. We will leave the wound open and repack it with gauze until it heals from the bottom up, inside-to-out. It's going to take about six weeks to heal completely, but it's the best way to overcome the infection. We'll advance the drain day by day until it's out, and we'll change the packing three times a day to remove any pus or bacteria that accumulate as healing proceeds. We also will keep Mr. Gulliver on antibiotics for the next seven to ten days.

***

When Mr. Gulliver has been transferred out of the operating room and into the Post Anesthesia Recovery Room, I return to the medical school library to search for a topic I can talk about at Grand Rounds—retained foreign bodies. The data are sparse—nobody is eager to publish their mistakes—but it makes for fascinating reading. Although I cannot tell him, I feel as though I should thank Mr. Gulliver for providing me a topic for my upcoming grand rounds.

I learn that most retained foreign bodies become covered by a sterile capsule and, remarkably, many do not cause symptoms. Many are extruded out of the body, often through a wound. Some erode slowly into the intestine and are expelled into the toilet with the stool. This may take months or even years to occur.

Some retained sponges become infected, similar to what occurred in Mr. Gulliver, but this usually occurs within a few years of surgery. Forty years, Mr. Gulliver's experience is most unusual and was almost certainly caused by his dental work. I am eager to see what bacteria will be recovered from Mr. Gulliver's blood and the extracted sponge, and see if they match those normally found in the mouth. But it will take several days for the cultures to grow out.

The medico-legal issues of this case also are interesting. They vary from state to state, but in most cases the legal liability is two years. Certainly 40 years far exceeds the liability of the surgeon. Who knows if the surgeon who was responsible for this case is even alive after all this time?

In any case, I think I have a topic for Grand Rounds, "Retained Foreign Body", and no one will know as much about it as I will, not even Lenny. When I tell Lenny about our patient, he shrugs indifferently.

"See?" he says. "You were worried about finding a subject for Grand Rounds. I told you it would be a piece of cake."

CHAPTER 38

INSTITUTIONAL REVIEW BOARD (IRB)

INTEROFFICE MEMO B

From: Dennis Halvorsen, MD, PhD, Associate Dean for Research and Chairman, University Institutional Review Board (IRB)

To: Senior Surgical Resident

Dear Doctor,

We are pleased to invite you to attend the monthly meeting of the University Institutional Review Board (IRB). This committee evaluates all proposals submitted by clinical faculty who wish to perform research involving human subjects. The purpose of the committee is to protect human subjects.

The IRB also determines whether patients have been adequately informed regarding the risks and benefits of participating in a given study.

***

So, I ask myself, do I want to go to this meeting? The answer is No-o-o, I do not. It sounds like just another boring meeting. On the other hand, I have a strong interest in clinical research. I know what I'll do; I'll prepare an escape route. I'll have Chris Gabel page me at one o'clock. If the meeting is unbearable, I'll excuse myself; if it's interesting, I'll stick around. Either way, there's free food (Whoever said there's no free lunch?)

***

The IRB meets monthly in the Dean's Conference Room, a crowded, windowless chamber where 13 people are crammed into a space fit for 10. Everyone sits around a long rosewood table, with the committee composed of representatives of active clinical departments that perform clinical research

Dr. Halvorsen, Chairman of the IRB Committee, sits at the head of the table, directly opposite me. A short man with an intense gaze and a crooked cigarette-stained smile sits in a wheelchair beside him.

"Ivan Kabelefsky," he says as he thrusts his hand over the table toward me. "I'm Kabelefsky," he says again with a strong Russian accent. "From Pharmacology." His palm is damp and as oily as a can of sardines.

A bulky gentleman in a white lab coat sitting next to Kabelefsky also reaches across the table. "Welcome," he says, jutting forth a powerful jaw. "Gerhart Ganz from Neurology."

"Walter Hartwig from Radiology," a florid, heavy set man says, offering his hand as well.

I introduce myself as a senior resident in General Surgery.

"What brings you here?" Dr. Hartwig asks politely.

"I was invited," I say. "To learn about the Institutional Review Board. I have an interest in basic and clinical research."

Everyone at the table expresses their encouragement.

"Very good," Dr. Hartwig says. "I'm sure you will learn a lot here. You may not believe it when you hear our discussions, but we are all friends. "Right, Kabelefsky?"

"Right," Kabelefsky responds, but his hand is raised to cover his face, and I cannot decipher his expression.

***

"Twelve o'clock," Dr. Halvorsen announces, "Time to get started."

Everyone sets their lunch sandwich aside, grabs a can of soda pop, and drags their stack of documents to within easy reach on the rosewood table.

There is much shuffling of papers as we extract our multi-page agendas from the foot-high stack of documents that had been sent to us for this meeting. Halvorsen's secretary sits behind him, receiving and returning documents over his shoulder as fast as he can read and scrawl his signature on them.

"The first protocol," Halvorsen says. "requires only Expedited Review. It offers negligible risk."

"Protocol number Twelve-ENT, it compares two well-established antihistamine agents in their ability to block excess nasal secretions. There are no new agents used in this study, and the doses employed are equal to those currently sold over the counter. Assignment of treatments will be randomized, and neither the patients nor the caregivers will know which medication they have been given. This study is funded by one of the companies supplying the medications. I assume you all have read the protocol."

I did not bother to read it, but I'm not about to advertise that fact. I keep my head down. Besides, I'm not sure anyone cares what a visiting fireman like me thinks about this protocol. It certainly seems harmless enough.

"Are there any questions? "Halvorsen asks. He looks around the room "If not, do I hear a motion?"

"Move to accept," Dr. Hartwig says.

"Good." All hands are raised in approval.

Dr. Halvorsen continues. "The next protocol, MED-twenty-seven, is from Cardiology. It requires a formal review, not a low-risk Expedited Review. It is concerned with methods of treatment with one of two drugs in patients who have atrial fibrillation.

These patients are currently receiving Coumadin, an anticoagulant, and all patients will be assigned to receive a placebo control drug or active medication in addition to anticoagulant medication. The protocol will be presented by Dr. Eddington from the Department of Medicine.

Dr. Eddington hunches forward over the rosewood table, and presents the technical details of the protocol.

His presentation is thorough and informative. Several members of the IRB ask questions about the relative risks of the drugs that are to be used. "The object of the proposed clinical protocol," Eddington says. "is to compare the efficacy of the two drugs while minimizing the risk of bleeding, nausea or other complications."

I have to admit it; this heady stuff is unexpectedly interesting, from a research point of view, and also in its application to daily clinical practice. In fact, we have two patients on our service now who are receiving Coumadin for atrial fibrillation.

One youthful-looking member of the IRB raises his hand. It is Dr. Mahaney, a lean nattily-dressed member of a department called Clinical Pharmacology. It is a well-funded division of the Department of Medicine.

After asking several questions about the pharmacology, Dr. Mahaney turns his attention to statistical issues. This unleashes a fire storm from Dr. Kabelefsky. An energized Kabelefsky tilts forward, almost propelling himself out of his wheelchair. He raises his Russian-accented voice to defend the proposed statistical methods to be employed.

"There is no assumption of normal distributions here," Kabelefsky says.

"These are nonparametric measures." Mahaney says.

"So?" Kabelefsky answers.

I have no idea what they are arguing about, but the others present in the room nod, implying that they understand. After a brief flurry of differing opinions, Drs. Mahaney and Kabelefsky sit back in their seats. The two men glare at each other, growling under their breaths. Each of them sits with the fingers of their left and right hands locked so tightly that their digits blanch. The two men remind me of a pair of conflict-ready roosters eager to do battle. I get the feeling that these two members of the committee are long-standing adversaries disagreeing at every turn. In fact, I think they hate each other. I can't help but wonder how they get anything done.

Taking advantage of a rare, uncontested moment, Dr. Halvorsen tries to recapture control of his meeting. "Any concerns regarding the Informed Consent?"

Tempers explode again as Kabelefsky and Mahaney wrangle over differences in the wording of the Informed Consent.

"I knew I shouldn't have asked," Halvorsen says loud enough for all of us to hear.

Finally, Mahaney and Kabelefsky sit back in their seats where they grumble and grouse restlessly. After a few minutes, the two protagonists stare at each other, sitting like innocent children with their hands folded in front of them, but they lean forward ready for action.

"All right," Halvorsen says. "Do I hear a motion?"

"Move approval," Dr. Ganz says.

"Further discussion?" Halvorsen asks.

"There is none," he says. In spite of the skirmish, the proposal wins unanimous approval. How could they do that? Be ready to kill each other one minute, yet vote unanimously in favor of the contested proposal the next.

Clearly, the Institutional Review Board acts as a watchdog for all sorts of research involving human subjects at the medical center. But from the emotions exhibited here, it is evident that Kabelefsky and Mahaney are deeply invested in the validity of the science, as well as the safety of the participants.

The meeting grinds on as Dr. Halvorsen announces the next research protocol offered by the Department of Radiology. "Rad-C28 is from Radiology. Dr. Hartwig will give the presentation."

Dr. Hartwig proceeds with a nervous routine that would make a professional baseball player proud when he steps up to the plate. Hartwig scratches his forehead, clears his throat, rubs his neck and prepares to speak, then he goes through it all over again. After two or three such rehearsals, he begins his presentation. "As we all know, intravenous contrast material can cause rashes, hives and other allergic reactions. In the present proposal, the investigators argue that *all* patients who receive intravenous contrast material of any sort should be given a one-time low dose of corticosteroids."

This proposal causes an instantaneous uproar as each member of the IRB argues in favor of, or against, the proposal, even though the proposal has not yet been presented. Everyone has an opinion, and no one seems capable of withholding it.

"Corticosteroids are not without their side effects," someone shouts.

"More patients will be harmed than helped," someone argues.

"If so few patients develop a reaction to contrast media, how many patients will we have to injure with corticosteroids to avoid a rare reaction to contrast media?" another voice asks.

An academic nurse, i.e., a clinical professor in the School of Nursing, articulates her concerns above the din of the IRB. She raises her voice, and then raises it again. Hers is a shrill utterance that can be heard in every surrounding county, and she will not be dissuaded from expressing her opinion. "This is dangerous," she says.

What is this all about? I ask myself. University politics? Research funding issues? Patient safety? Unlike the room full of true believers, I cannot keep myself from laughing. In just a few seconds everyone in the room is laughing, but the calm does not last for long.

In the midst of all this turmoil, my pager goes off.

"Call Chris Gabel, In the ER." It sounds like my opportunity to escape. But I'm not sure that I want to go. I make my way around the rosewood table and squeeze between two corpulent members of the committee. The phone is on the wall, just outside the conference room, next to the doorway. After some polite pushing, I finally get to the phone. One of my feet is in the hall where I'm listening to a telephone presentation about a patient in the ER. It sounds like appendicitis. My other foot is in the conference room where I am witnessing an intellectual battle over the questionable use of corticosteroids. I

stand straddling the threshold, facing two different problems at once. Unfortunately, I don't think I know enough yet about either issue to make a definitive decision.

Dr. Halvorsen looks up as I get off the phone. "Trouble?" he asks.

"I have to go. But this has been very informative. I'm looking forward to attending next month's meeting."

"Good," he says. "We'll be looking for you. In fact," he adds. "You should attend the Pharmacy and Therapeutics Committee also. In that committee we struggle with the use and cost of medications. Many of the same players here are on that committee."

"No thanks," I say. "I'm not sure how many of these Armageddons I could take."

Dr. Halvorsen laughs. "Oh, you will get used to them,"

So there I am, walking down the hall, half-way between the ER and the IRB office to see a patient with signs and symptoms of acute surgical illness. The IRB office and the ER are at opposite ends of the same building, and right now they couldn't be farther apart. I make a note to myself to call Dr. Halvorsen's secretary to find out who won the corticosteroid controversy. But first, I must see the patient in the Emergency Room. As I walk down the hall, I think of the life I am planning for myself, having a career in both clinical surgery and research. Can anyone be really good at two careers at a once?

CHAPTER 39

AT NIGHT, ALONE

It is one o'clock in the morning, and I am sitting up in bed in the Intensive Care Unit, unable to sleep. After serving almost twenty-five years as a doctor, medical administrator, teacher, and a scientific investigator, today I am a patient. Three weeks ago I learned that I have a rapidly enlarging thoracic aortic aneurysm, a dangerous lesion in the chest. Repair will require replacement of both the aorta and the overstretched aortic valve.

I think of Mr. Grant, the professor of mechanical engineering upon whom we operated when I was a first year resident. He had the same problem as I do, and he sailed through the operation. So why shouldn't I?

It's three a.m., and I cannot sleep. I hear Ernie delivering linens around hospital. "Hey mon, how's eva body doin?" His irritating chatter is unmistakable at this late hour. Remarkably, he's still here after all these years.

It's four a.m., and I've still had no sleep. Two of the ICU nurses are outside my room arguing about when to administer pre-op antibiotics. Their voices are not particularly loud, but I can hear every word they say. Don't they realize they're keeping everyone in the ICU awake? Maybe they are not keeping everyone awake, just me.

Five a.m. Who walks into my room, but Mrs. Greer? She's been the night nurse supervisor at the University

Hospital for as long as I can remember. She stops in to wish me luck. "As you know, you were scheduled to be the first case in the morning, but unfortunately, you're going to be delayed for about an hour and a half. The cardiac surgeons had a cardiac emergency, and they've been up all night trying to get him off the bypass pump.

"That's all I know," Mrs. Greer says. "But we'll keep you and your wife informed if anything changes."

How useful, I think to myself. That will give me an extra hour and a half of pre-op worrying time.

Six-thirty a.m. A Transportation Department orderly arrives to take me to the Operating Room. I'm glad he's here at last, but now, faced with the reality of it, I'm not so eager to go. Of course, I have no choice. He transfers me to a gurney, and then wheels me from the ICU to the operating room. As we roll through the hall, he tries to make small talk about the local sports teams, but I have no interest. We're through the swinging door to the Operating room and into Room Four, the heart surgery room.

As I slide off the gurney and onto the operating table, I hear the assuring voice of Dr. Hakeem, the Chief of Anesthesia. "I stay with you all day, however long it takes. But first we start with pre-op medication."

The operating room is unusually quiet for this hour of the morning, silent but for the hiss of oxygen. Pre-op intravenous medications are already swirling through my veins, and the world around me is becoming distant and disconnected; even the familiar hiss of the oxygen seems to be fading into the distance. I'm lying on my back with an ill-fitting oxygen mask pressing against my cheek.

"Forget those old masks," a familiar voice says. "Try one of these new ones. They are supposed to be more comfortable.

"There," he says. "Much better—a piece of cake."

SOME FINAL THOUGHTS...

EPILOGUE

NEW TECHNIQUES OF NON-INVASIVE DIAGNOSIS

The episodes described here occurred in the 1970s and 1980s. Many diagnostic and therapeutic techniques have developed since that time. The following describes some of the most noteworthy.

In the last 30 years, basic scientists have developed highly accurate noninvasive imaging techniques for visualizing anatomic structures. These methods include Computerized Tomography (CAT) scans and Nuclear Magnetic Resonance (NMR), technologies that are useful to health care providers in all fields of medicine.

NEW TECHNIQUES OF SURGERY

The last 30 years also has seen many changes in the practice and teaching of surgery. Of these, perhaps the most dramatic is the appearance of laparoscopy. This is a method for performing "minimally invasive" surgery through slender tubes. These include:

- Cholecystectomy (removal of the gall bladder)
- Appendectomy (removal of the appendix)
- Hiatal hernia
- Colectomy (removal of part of the large bowel)
- Splenectomy (removal of the spleen)
- Adrenalectomy, removal of the adrenal gland
- Nephrectomy for kidney transplant

- Bariatric surgery of the stomach for treatment of morbid obesity.
- Coronary artery by-pass
- Peripheral vascular surgery

And I'm sure there will be more to come. Use of these techniques has fulfilled demands of informed patients and is made possible by the aggressive development of methods and apparatus by manufacturers of new technologies.

NEW METHODS OF BOARD CERTIFICATION

In an attempt to achieve improved methods of certification the American Board of Surgery is developing a system of improved methods. This consists of four parts:

1. Evidence of professional standing as demonstrated by possession of an unrestricted medical license and appropriate hospital privileges,
2. Evidence of life-long learning and self-assessment with approval of practice validation,
3. Evidence of cognitive expertise, and
4. Evaluation of performance as measured by patient outcomes. Fulfillment of these continuous demands on skills, knowledge and performance will be evaluated by the Board in three-year cycles.

When a candidate initially seeks certification he or she will be expected to manage: a) 25 cases of Advanced Cardiac Life Support, b) 25 cases of Advanced Trauma Life Support, and c) will be exposed to the fundamentals of laparoscopic surgical techniques.

A final issue of concern to the Board is relevant to the number of hours worked by residents in training. Graduate medical education often requires trainees to work long hours. In order to protect both the fatigued trainee and the patients, the Accreditation Council for Graduate Medical Education (ACGME) determined that resident's duties should be limited to an 80-hour work week. In addition, the ACGME insisted that on duty periods longer than 16 hours include a 5 hour uninterrupted period of continuous sleep between 10 p.m. and 8 a.m.

However, even if vigorously followed, the ACGME and Institute of Medicine (IOM) are struggling with three unsolved problems:

1. Finding the trained personnel to do the work currently performed by the residents,
2. Finding a way to pay for this additional trained staff, and
3. Devising systems that will provide smooth transition when one resident leaves and another comes on to assume responsibility for care of a patient. Remarkably, use of these shorter work hours has not yet proven to be clinically beneficial.

Made in the USA
Lexington, KY
08 March 2012